Integrated Science

Volume 29

The **Integrated Science** Series aims to publish the most relevant and novel research in all areas of Formal Sciences, Physical and Chemical Sciences, Biological Sciences, Medical Sciences, and Social Sciences. We are especially focused on the research involving the integration of two of more academic fields offering an innovative view, which is one of the main focuses of Universal Scientific Education and Research Network (USERN), science without borders.

Integrated Science is committed to upholding the integrity of the scientific record and will follow the Committee on Publication Ethics (COPE) guidelines on how to deal with potential acts of misconduct and correcting the literature.

Sara Spowart
Editor

Global Happiness and Humanitarian Assistance

Systemic Solutions

Springer

Editor
Sara Spowart
University of South Florida
Saint Petersburg, FL, USA

ISSN 2662-9461 ISSN 2662-947X (electronic)
Integrated Science
ISBN 978-3-031-71788-8 ISBN 978-3-031-71789-5 (eBook)
https://doi.org/10.1007/978-3-031-71789-5

This Springer imprint is published by the registered company Springer Nature Switzerland AG
The registered company address is: Gewerbestrasse 11, 6330 Cham, Switzerland

Contents

Part I

Looking at the Big Picture

Introduction and Overview

1

Sara Spowart

Abstract

This section provides an introduction and overview of the importance of investigating happiness in the context of global health. Since COVID-19 issues such as depression, anxiety, addiction, and chronic disease have been rising issues worldwide. It has become increasingly important to adopt interventions such as mindfulness, Cognitive Behavior Therapy, and Rational Behavior Therapy to address the rising levels of mental illness, addiction, and chronic illness for global health. The remaining chapters in this book are an exploration of case studies, worldwide phenomena, and policy options for improving happiness and well-being on a global scale.

Keywords

Global health • Mental illness • COVID-19 • Mindfulness • Family health

1 Introduction and Overview

Understanding what helps us to be happy and what causes unhappiness is increasingly important as the rates of depression, anxiety, mental illness, addiction, and chronic disease are on the rise worldwide. The World Health Organization states that there is a 25.6% increase in anxiety and a 27.6% increase in depression worldwide. Since the COVID-19 pandemic, there has been an 11% rise in suicide rates and 20% rise in trauma and stress. Furthermore, approximately one in four Americans between the ages of 18–24 years have considered suicide in the last month

S. Spowart (✉)
University of South Florida, Tampa, FL, USA
e-mail: compassionbasedhappiness@gmail.com

S. Spowart (ed.), *Global Happiness and Humanitarian Assistance*, Integrated Science 29, https://doi.org/10.1007/978-3-031-71789-5_1

and suffer from some degree of suicidal ideation (World Health Organization, 2022; Vahratian et al., 2021). This increase in mental illness is in many ways related to the COVID pandemic and the multitude of factors that accompanied the pandemic such as increased levels of isolation and loneliness; new types of relationship, work, school, and life stress; as well as significant increases in domestic violence, and economic stressors with unemployment and inflation. There were negative impacts on relationships, finances, and everyday life functioning due to the COVID pandemic. These negative impacts are ongoing as we still recover from the aftermath. For many families, this means managing the long-term negative impacts of inflation, illness, child trauma from at-home isolation, relationship and work stress, and how the world has changed since the pandemic (World Health Organization, 2022; Vahratian et al., 2021).

Women and children have experienced worse mental health impacts than men globally as a result of the pandemic. The increasing gender pay gap, worldwide inflation, heightened childcare and household responsibilities inordinately placed on women and worsened domestic violence levels all contribute to mental illness (World Health Organization, 2022; Vahratian et al., 2021). The rates for mental illness were significantly higher for women than men in the pre-pandemic era; however, the pandemic greatly exasperated this and worsened the prevalence of this divide. COVID altered the way that relationships occurred from dating, family events, children's friendships, and the stress on domestic partnerships. Weddings were moved to online streaming, dating was largely through online video interactions, children were subjected to much more screen time and interacting with friends through multiplayer online games, and domestic partnerships were strained as partners spent isolated time together in one household (World Health Organization, 2022; Vahratian et al., 2021). This isolation and new way of interaction helped to improve and focus on the family more but also put more strain on already existing issues. It highlighted a lot of underlying issues that already existed in families and interpersonal relationships because of forced isolation and seclusion from others. Previously existing discontent and issues that may have been under the surface and ignored for years or decades, could no longer be ignored with the isolation and stressors that occurred. The stressors exasperated underlying issues and brought out the reality of familial unhappiness and interpersonal relationships that had been put on the back burner. Therapists saw record numbers in individuals seeking and needing therapy and mental health treatment as their interpersonal relationship issues were exasperated and could no longer be ignored (World Health Organization, 2022; Vahratian et al., 2021).

In particular, the family unit and relationships were impacted due to extra stressors. The experience of isolation from other support networks due to COVID restrictions and quarantines, working and studying from home created a new dynamic that put additional stress on many relationships. Family members and individuals living in the same home tended to have additional pressure placed on relationships due to increased amounts of interaction and time spent in the same living environment. Also, other previously used outlets for stress and interaction were largely not available due to COVID and so it was common for individuals to feel isolated from friends and other previously used stress outlets. For this reason, greater stress was placed on live-in relationships, as well as unhealthy coping mechanisms such as excess food and alcohol consumption as well as different forms of addiction. Underlying mental health and relational concerns were exasperated amongst families as individuals were forced to function in isolation from home, cut off from their previous stress outlets. Our closest relationships are some of the most critical variables for our happiness and therefore the heightened stress and dysfunction that resulted from COVID policies resulted in significant declines in happiness due to relational challenges. This was also evidenced by the heightened levels of domestic violence and abuse during COVID in the United States and many other countries worldwide due to quarantine and COVID-related restrictions (World Health Organization, 2022; Vahratian et al., 2021).

The heightened levels of mental illness worldwide point to the importance of improving well-being and happiness to counteract this growing concern. To address this need for well-being improvement it is important to identify factors that impact our happiness levels. Important aspects that influence happiness are mindfulness, self-compassion, non-judgment, diet, connection, and positive perspective (Coo & Salanova, 2018; Ortet et al., 2020). Mindfulness is the practice of paying attention to your mind and its contents in the present moment in a non-reactive, non-judgmental manner. Mindfulness meditation is the formal exercise of promoting greater awareness of the present moment so that it can be applied to everyday life (Coo & Salanova, 2018; Ortet et al., 2020). There has been considerable attention to mindfulness studies and their impact on reducing symptoms of psychological disorders and somatic illness. However, insufficient focus has been given to Mindfulness-Based Interventions (MBIs) as a way to improve well-being, and increase compassion, self-care, positive affect and happiness (Coo & Salanova, 2018; Ortet et al., 2020).

Mindfulness is positively associated with increased energy, life satisfaction, and interpersonal relationships (Coo & Salanova, 2018; Ortet et al., 2020). There are opportunities for applying mindfulness meditation to increase and cultivate adaptive behavior and positive states of mind. Due to the prior focus on reducing the negative, there is a substantial gap in the academic literature on the positive impacts of mindfulness practices (Coo & Salanova, 2018; Ortet et al., 2020). The work of Coo and Salanova (2018) and Ortet et al. (2020), points to the application of mindfulness in a workplace setting as a way to increase work engagement, positivity, and feeling in the state of flow. However, in general, there are applications for cultivating happiness and transforming and focusing on positive mental states. It can also be applied to help create greater awareness of positive characteristics of one's life and focus on creating more positivity (Coo & Salanova, 2018; Ortet et al., 2020).

Through practices like Cognitive Behavior Therapy and Rational Emotive Behavior Therapy, thoughts and beliefs can be reframed and geared towards a more positive, optimistic, 'happy' perspective (Ellis, 2021). Cognitive behavioral therapy (CBT) encourages one to become aware and challenge the validity, of their innate cognitive processes (Beck & Fernandez, 1998). Through such awareness, one can distinguish healthy from unhealthy thoughts, realize how thoughts control mood, affect, and behavior, and then incorporate healthy self-statements. According to Beck and Fernandez (1998) CBT is almost always structured into three stages: (1) cognitive preparation, (2) acquiring the skills needed to cope and change behavior, and (3) applying the skills to real-life situations. Cognitive preparation and skill acquisition consists of, but is not limited to, clients identifying items and thoughts that may precipitate an irrational response and developing a system of coping mechanisms like cognitive reframing and relaxation practices, to help establish appropriate reactions and interventions. Originally, CBT was used to treat aggressive behaviors and anger; however, many therapists have realized that CBT can enhance the effectiveness of treatment for varying disorders across the mental health spectrum (Beck & Fernandez, 1998). Large effect sizes have been found for the treatment of depression, anxiety, trauma and children's mental illness (Butler et al., 2006).

Rational Emotive Behavioral Therapy (REBT) is a subcategory practice of CBT (Dobson, 2009). Specifically, REBT is distinct in that it is a type of psychotherapy that encourages clients to question their belief systems. It teaches clients that they have control over their feelings while encouraging non-judgment toward oneself and others. REBT is highly cognitive and discipline-oriented and relies on direct action and homework. REBT often involves journaling, meditation, and mindfulness as tools to help one overcome personal obstacles (Ellis, 2008). REBT also teaches clients to remain calm when faced with situations that lead to negative emotions and to not allow emotions to be self-destructive. Professionals using REBT techniques encourage their clients to practice in everyday situations the strategies taught within the therapeutic environment, thus helping clients to become more understanding of themselves. Through the use of REBT practices, clients learn to become more skeptical thinkers and begin to question their behavior and ideas, thus altering the harmful tendencies they are trying to overcome. In REBT, the emphasis is on the control one has over his/her thoughts and emotions within a philosophy of unconditional acceptance. REBT can be applied to help individuals understand how their environment, family, society and circumstances are impacting them. Through this approach, not only can a client investigate their own negative beliefs that are adversely affecting them, but it is also possible to understand family, societal, cultural, and environmental beliefs that are hurting someone (Ellis, 2008).

References

Beck, R., & Fernandez, E. (1998). Cognitive-behavioral therapy in the treatment of anger: A meta-analysis. *Cognitive Therapy and Research, 22*(1), 63–74.

Butler, A. C., Chapman, J. E., Forman, E. M., & Beck, A. T. (2006). The empirical status of cognitive behavioral therapy: A review of meta-analyses. *Clinical Psychology Review, 26*(1), 17–31.

Coo, C., & Salanova, M. (2018). Mindfulness can make you happy-and-productive: A mindfulness-controlled trial and its effects on happiness, work engagement, and performance. *Journal of Happiness Studies, 19*(6), 1691–1711.

Dobson, K. S. (Ed.). (2009). *Handbook of cognitive-behavioral therapies*. Guilford Press.

Ellis, A. (2008). 6 Rational emotive behavior therapy. In Feltham, C. (Ed) *Which psychotherapy* (pp. 51–67). California, US: Sage Publications.

Ellis, D. J. (2021). The power and compassion of rational emotive behavior therapy (REBT). In *Research anthology on rehabilitation practices and therapy* (pp. 1354–1365). IGI Global.

Ortet, G., Pinazo, D., Walker, D., Gallego, S., Mezquita, L., & Ibáñez, M. I. (2020). Personality and nonjudging make you happier: Contribution of the Five-Factor Model, mindfulness facets and a mindfulness intervention to subjective well-being. *PloS one, 15*(2), e0228655.

Vahratian, A., Blumberg, S. J., Terlizzi, E. P., & Schiller, J. S. (2021). Symptoms of anxiety or depressive disorder and use of mental health care among adults during the COVID-19 pandemic—United States, August 2020–February 2021. *Morbidity and Mortality Weekly Report, 70*(13), 490.

World Health Organization. (2022). *World mental health report: Transforming mental health for all.*

Examining the Influence of Sustainable Development Goals (SDG) on Happiness: A Systems Thinking Perspective

2

Anthony J. Masys

Abstract

The topic of happiness has gained significant attention during the last decade. With the influx of popular books and research into the topic of happiness, our understanding of the 'emergence' of happiness and its significance and connection to well-being is increasing. 'International institutions, national governments and communities are promoting and measuring happiness in various ways' (Iriarte and Musikanski, International Journal of Community Well-Being 1:115–135, 2019:115). The General Assembly of the United Nations in 2012 proclaimed 20 March the International Day of Happiness (UN DESA). This was predated in 1972 with the declaration by 4th King of Bhutan, King Jigme Singye Wangchuck that 'Gross National Happiness is more important than Gross Domestic Product'. Recognizing the emphasis on a more holistic approach towards progress in personnel and national well-being, this chapter employs a system thinking and complexity lens in the examination of the extant literature and data on happiness and well-being and presents an 'interpretive' network analysis revealing the inherent relationality and influence of various factors on the emergence of happiness. The insights are far reaching in terms of recognizing the influence of public policy objectives pertaining to the Sustainable Development Goals (SDG) on national happiness.

Keywords

Happiness • Systems thinking • SDG • Social determinants

A. J. Masys (✉)
University of South Florida, Tampa, FL, USA
e-mail: tmasys@usf.edu

S. Spowart (ed.), *Global Happiness and Humanitarian Assistance*, Integrated Science 29, https://doi.org/10.1007/978-3-031-71789-5_2

1 Introduction

The COVID-19 pandemic certainly stress-tested societal systems resulting in an awakening to the fragility that resides within our national and global communities (UNDRR & UNU-EHS, 2022). Of note is the toll the pandemic had on health-care workers exacerbating workplace stress and burnout in health settings. As reported in Murthy (2022:577) 'More than half of health workers report symptoms of burnout, and many are contending with insomnia, depression, anxiety, post-traumatic stress disorder, or other mental health challenges.' The WHO (2022) reports that during the first year of the pandemic '...global prevalence of anxiety and depression increased by a massive 25%'. It is further reported (WHO, 2022) that '...one major explanation for the increase is the unprecedented stress caused by the social isolation resulting from the pandemic. Linked to this were constraints on people's ability to work, seek support from loved ones and engage in their communities...Loneliness, fear of infection, suffering and death for oneself and for loved ones, grief after bereavement and financial worries have also all been cited as stressors leading to anxiety and depression'.

Emotional well-being is also reported as directly or indirectly being implicated in some of the '...world's biggest killers: heart disease, obesity, hypertension, tobacco-related diseases such as cancer, suicide, and conditions related to alcohol dependency and binge drinking' (Harvard, ND). Further, Harvard (ND) reports that '...research involving representative samples of 95 percent of the world's population suggests that "emotions matter to health everywhere." The emotion-health connection is not unique to certain countries, regions, or levels of economic development'.

The WHO (2021:10) defines well-being as:

> '...a positive state experienced by individuals and societies. Similar to health, it is a resource for daily life and is determined by social, economic and environmental conditions. Well-being encompasses quality of life, as well as the ability of people and societies to contribute to the world in accordance with a sense of meaning and purpose. Focusing on wellbeing supports the tracking of the equitable distribution of resources, overall thriving, and sustainability. A society's well-being can be observed by the extent to which they are resilient, build capacity for action, and are prepared to transcend challenges.'

The topic of happiness has gained significant attention during the last decade. With popular books and research into the topic of happiness our understanding of the 'emergence' of happiness and its significance and connection to well-being is increasing. Since 2012 'The *World Happiness Report'* a publication of the Sustainable Development Solutions Network has provided a global analysis of happiness by country (WHR). Similarly, there has been significant research investigating the societal determinants of happiness such as the recent contribution of Araki (2023:1) which examined evidence from 152 countries over a 15-year period. Interestingly, research examining the SDG and Happiness metrics proposes an Aggregated Happiness Index (AHI) to bridge the gap (Iriarte et al., 2019:115).

Recognizing the emphasis on a holistic approach towards progress in personnel and national well-being, this chapter employs a system thinking lens in the examination of the extant literature and data on happiness and well-being and presents an 'interpretive' network analysis revealing the inherent relationality and influence of various factors on the emergence of happiness. The insights are far reaching in terms of recognizing the influence of public policy objectives pertaining to the Sustainable Development Goals (SDG) and national happiness. What is not examined and beyond the scope of this chapter is the 'tipping point' pertaining to the emergence of happiness stemming from the influence of various factors. Further data driven research would be required to examine this area.

1.1 Happiness and Well-Being

The importance of happiness and well-being at the individual and national level is of significant research interest that is certainly rooted in the public and global health domain. The complexity inherent within the experience (or emergence) of happiness is expressed by Martin Seligman noted in Theobald and Cooper (2012:17) as '...a matrix of interwoven factors which combine in a unique way to bring about our emotional state'. The Cambridge Dictionary defines well-being as the state of being healthy and happy.

Nemati and Maralan (2016:194) present happiness as a multi-dimensional construct influenced by a number of significant factors ranging from our internal experience to the exterior realities in which we live in affecting our well-being. The complexity and emergent nature of happiness is well argued in Badri et al., (2022: 3). A compendium of definitions pertaining to happiness are well articulated in Medvedev et al., (2018:2–4). As described in Medvedev et al., (2018:1), '...the existing definitions of happiness, subjective well-being, and health related quality of life and the main components assigned to these constructs in the research literature suggest conceptual overlap between these dimensions.' In this paper we present a complexity view of the 'emergence of happiness' that leverages some of the key features from complexity theory.

The construct of happiness gained a significant recognition when the phrase 'gross national happiness' was first coined by the 4th King of Bhutan, King Jigme Singye Wangchuck, in 1972 when he declared, "Gross National Happiness is more important than Gross Domestic Product". This bold stance certainly established a connection between sustainable development and national well-being. In so doing, Bhutan developed and operationalized the Gross National Happiness Index (GNH) to include '...both traditional areas of socio-economic concern such as living standards, health and education and less traditional aspects of culture and psychological wellbeing. It is a holistic reflection of the general wellbeing of the Bhutanese population rather than a subjective psychological ranking of 'happiness' alone'. In establishing the index, Bhutan identified 9 domains (Table 1) and 33 indicators to support their analysis.

Table 1 GNH index includes nine domains

Psychological wellbeing
Health
Education
Time use
Cultural diversity and resilience
Good governance
Community vitality
Ecological diversity and resilience
Living standards

The World Happiness Report (WHR) has been published since 2012. This stems from the sponsored UN Resolution "Happiness: Towards a holistic approach to development," adopted by the General Assembly of the United Nations on 19 July 2011. As described at (WHR) '…the resolution invited national governments to give more importance to happiness and well-being in determining how to achieve and measure social and economic development'. As cited in Araki (2023:1) and derived from the World Happiness Reports (Helliwell et al. 2020, 2021, 2022, 2023) the complexity of factors and influence on the emergence of happiness points to '…six variables as the key country-level determinants of happiness: GDP per capita, social support, healthy life expectancy at birth, freedom to make life choices, generosity, and perceptions of corruption'. These reports provide the foundation of data sources for the network analysis.

1.2 Sustainable Development Goals (SDGs)

The UN Sustainable Development Goals (SDGs) were adopted in 2015 as part of a 2030 Sustainability Agenda. The 2030 Sustainable Development Agenda is comprised of 17 Sustainable Development Goals (SDGs), 169 targets and 232 indicators, with an ambition to establish a "plan of action for people, planet and prosperity" (UN SDG) within a timeframe of 15 years (2015–2030). The 17 SDGs (Fig. 1) do not exist in a silo but are characterized by the complexity of the world we live in. As reported in WHO (2022b).

> 'The universality and interconnectedness of the SDGs is a core feature of the 2030 Agenda for Sustainable Development. It was designed in response to growing appreciation that simultaneous and complex adaptive factors affect development across sectors and established silos, and traverse different segments of society. The SDGs involve the entire world and are integrated and indivisible, balancing economic, social and environmental dimensions. Health and well-being are similarly determined by factors lying outside what is traditionally seen as the health sector: namely through the overlapping and intersectional social, structural, economic, political, environmental and commercial determinants of health'.

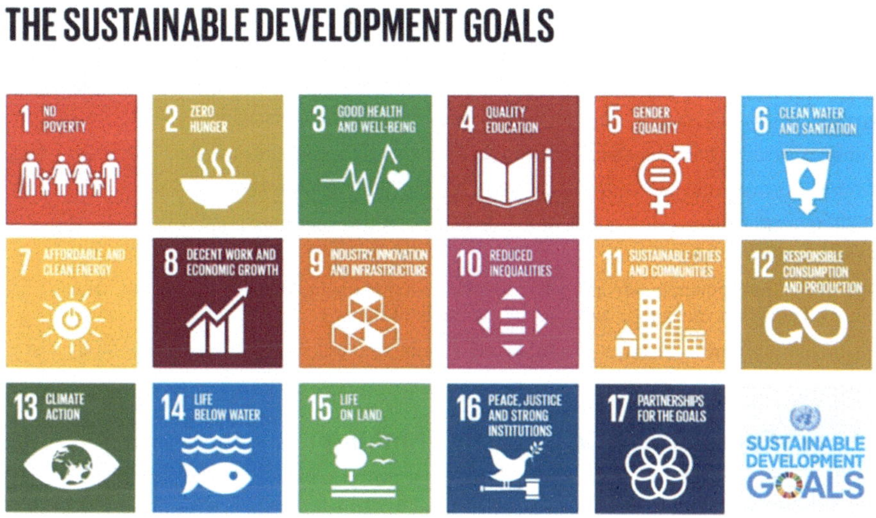
THE SUSTAINABLE DEVELOPMENT GOALS
1 NO POVERTY
2 ZERO HUNGER
3 GOOD HEALTH AND WELL-BEING
4 QUALITY EDUCATION
5 GENDER EQUALITY
6 CLEAN WATER AND SANITATION
7 AFFORDABLE AND CLEAN ENERGY
8 DECENT WORK AND ECONOMIC GROWTH
9 INDUSTRY, INNOVATION AND INFRASTRUCTURE
10 REDUCED INEQUALITIES
11 SUSTAINABLE CITIES AND COMMUNITIES
12 RESPONSIBLE CONSUMPTION AND PRODUCTION
13 CLIMATE ACTION
14 LIFE BELOW WATER
15 LIFE ON LAND
16 PEACE, JUSTICE AND STRONG INSTITUTIONS
17 PARTNERSHIPS FOR THE GOALS
SUSTAINABLE DEVELOPMENT GOALS

Fig. 1 Sustainable development goals (UN, 2015)

As reported in Sachs (2016:61), 'Happiness data offer a powerful new tool for examining alternative visions of human well-being... Sustainable Development advocates claim that the happiness is achieved through a multi-dimensional focus on economic, social, and environmental objectives. Here we examine the data collected from the WHR and using a thematic analysis connect the SDG to the Social Determinants of Happiness.

2 Discussion

As reported in Iriarte et al. (2019:115), 'International institutions, national governments and communities are promoting and measuring happiness in various ways. The groundbreaking work of Helliwell et al. (2020, 2021, 2022, 2023) through the World Happiness Report has documented the thought leadership and evidence to support a proposed social determinant of happiness and reveals the inherent complexity associated with happiness. Bringing a complexity lens to the analysis of happiness and linkages to SDG is apropos. Gentili, (2021) proposes the application of complexity science as it pertains to the SDGs. Similarly, Urry (2003) in his book 'Global Complexity' examines global processes and shows how ideas of chaos and complexity support our understanding of social order reframing our understanding from a linear event-based model to one embracing nonlinearity, interdependencies and interconnectivity. As cited in Masys (2023), '...The inherent interdependency and interconnectivity across the 17 SDG as detailed in (Coenen et al., 2022; Dawes, 2022; Laumann et al., 2022; Le Blanc, 2015) points to the requirement for a networked/ systems view of the SDG'.

Table 2 Key features of complex systems (Sweeney & Griffiths, 2002:2)

Complex systems consist of multiple components. Such systems are understood by observing the rich interaction of these components, not simply understanding the system's structure
The interaction between components can produce unpredictable behaviour
Complex systems have a history and are sensitive to initial conditions
Complex systems interact with and are influenced by their environment
The interactions between elements of the system are non-linear. Small inputs may have large effects, and vice versa
The interactions generate new properties, called emergent behaviours of the system, which cannot be explained through studying the elements of the system
In complex systems such emergent behaviour cannot be predicted

2.1 Complexity and Systems Thinking

The inherent features of complex systems of interdependencies and interconnectivity point to the emergence of new system properties. Informed by complexity theory, Ottino (2003:293) argues that 'complex systems cannot be understood by studying parts in isolation. The very essence of the system lies in the interaction between parts and the overall behavior that emerges from the interactions. This complexity lens challenges traditional notions of causality and assumptions of equilibrium. With this lens comes a new vocabulary and understanding regarding systems, providing a new set of concepts for describing complex nonlinear systems (Capra, 2005). Urry (2003) describes how complexity recognizes the emergent properties that result from the dynamic interaction within a system, thereby developing collective properties that are not reflected in the individual components. As noted in Styhre (2002), the complexity perspective recognizes that changes result from a multiplicity of interconnected causes and effects. The traditional linear perspective makes comprehension of the interrelationships difficult to conceive of.

Systems thinking, according to Senge (1990:68) 'is a discipline for seeing wholes. It is a framework for seeing interrelationships rather than things, for seeing patterns of change rather than static snapshots. Cilliers (1998:2) remarks that a complex system '…is not constituted merely by the sum of its components, but also by the intricate relationships between these components. In cutting up a system, the analytical method destroys what it seeks to understand'. In particular, complexity thinking has facilitated a new thinking about the concept of system and offered a new set of conceptual tools. Table 2 lists some of the key features of complex systems.

2.2 Analysis

Recognizing the emphasis on a holistic approach towards progress in personnel and national well-being, the analysis leveraged a complexity and systems thinking lens in the examination of the extant literature and data on happiness and well-being and presents an 'interpretive' network analysis revealing the inherent relationality and influence of various factors on the emergence of happiness. The features of a network are rooted in the relationality inherent in the interconnected nodes. Networks are constituted by nodes and edges or links. The power of the network representation is rooted in its common language, mathematical foundations, and data-driven computational methods (Barabasi, 2016; Easley & Kleinberg, 2010). As noted in (Weber et al., 2021) the networks represent complex and enduring connections stretching across time and space between peoples and things. This relationality provides insights into the dynamic nature of networks and in this case to the 'emergence' of happiness.

Urry (2003:24–25) describes the idea of emergence:

> '… There is a collective properties of all sorts of phenomena. …complexity examines how components of a system through their interaction spontaneously develop collective properties, even simple properties such as color…. thus the flavour of sugar is not present in the carbon, hydrogen and oxygen atoms that comprise it. These are all striking nonlinear consequences that are not present within or reducible to the very many individual components that comprise such activities.

Helliwell et al. (2020, 2021, 2022, 2023) advocate for six variables as the key country-level determinants of happiness: GDP per capita, social support, healthy life expectancy at birth, freedom to make life choices, generosity, and perceptions of corruption. The idea of the social determinants of happiness is not a stretch considering the social determinants of health.

As noted in the WHO Glossary of terms (WHO, 2021:32).

> The social determinants of health are the social, cultural, political, economic and environmental conditions in which people are born, grow up, live, work and age, and their access to power, decision-making, money and resources that give rise to these conditions of daily life. The social determinants of health influence a person's opportunity to be healthy, their risk of illness, health behaviours and healthy life expectancy.

Key in this definition is the word 'influence'. This 'influence' relates back to our discussion of the properties of complex systems in terms of nonlinear behaviour and emergence. The inherent interconnectivity of these variables with the SDGs is examined using GEPHI, a software visualization tool supporting network analysis. The data for this analysis is derived from the WHR and thematic analysis across the extant literature on happiness and SDGs.

As noted earlier, there has been significant research investigating the societal determinants of happiness such as the recent contribution of Araki (2023:1) which examined evidence from 152 countries over a 15-year period. Similarly, research examining the SDG and Happiness metrics proposes an Aggregated Happiness Index (AHI) to bridge the gap (Iriarte et al., 2019:115).

The inherent relationality and influence across the network structure comprised of nodes and edges, gives rise to emergent properties. Urry (2003: 24–25) characterizes emergence through the analogy of sugar whereby the flavour of sugar is not present in the carbon, hydrogen and oxygen atoms that comprise it. These are nonlinear consequences that are not present with the constituent parts. As noted in Gentili (2021:122) '...a more recent classification is based on the idea that Complex Systems can be represented as networks, and every type of network originates its peculiar emergent properties'. This points to the dynamic nature of systems with '...inherent interconnections, woven through overlapping relationships of causal effects that carry ripples of impacts from any system driver to any others, synergizing emergent phenomena beyond the sum of its components, and often through one or several degrees of feedback loops' (Fortier, 2020).

Figure 2 shows the network components (SDG and national happiness variables) and influence between them. Of note is the size of the SDGs. They have been scaled in a representation of their influence on the happiness variables. Similarly in Fig. 3, we show the effect of the SDGs on the happiness variables as a function of their centrality. The complexity lens sees the world, as in Figs. 2 and 3, as interconnected '...rich with forms and patterns that have been shaped by history and context' (Boulton et al., 2015:1). This is an important interpretive lens as it lends itself to better understanding of the dynamics of the network in terms of intervention strategies, influence and intended/unintended consequences. As argued in Boulton et al., (2015:9):

> 'Form is described as a patterning of relationships which sustains for a time. Form emerges from relationships between the things of which it is constituted. So this presents a view of the world as systemic, emergent, and co-created, rather than a view of the world as pre-fixed, predictable, and controllable'.

This is important to understand when it comes to policy makers and interventions amongst the SDGs. Boulton et al., (2015:126) notes that '...a complexity perspective will emphasize that whatever change we introduce will interact with what is already in place, and that the particular experiences, biases and histories...will play a part in influencing the outcomes of the change we introduce'. History matters. Context matters. Complex causality matters. Viewing happiness as an emergent property stemming from but not limited to the influences of the SDG, suggests that policy makers at the national scale should consider the 'weak signals' of change in happiness indicators to support sensemaking (Masys, 2021). Given the effect of the COVID-19 pandemic on global SDGs (UNDRR & UNU-EHS, 2022), the importance of understanding the dynamic nature and influences across the network gives rise to the criticality pertaining to the planning for and designing for resilience in the face of shocks. Embracing resilience thinking is an imperative for policy makers. Policy makers cannot be expected to anticipate all surprising shocks to a system, '...instead by encouraging adaptation, agility, cooperation, connectivity, and diversity, resilience thinking can bring a different way of being in the world, and to a deeper engagement with it' (Zolli & Healy, 2012:16).

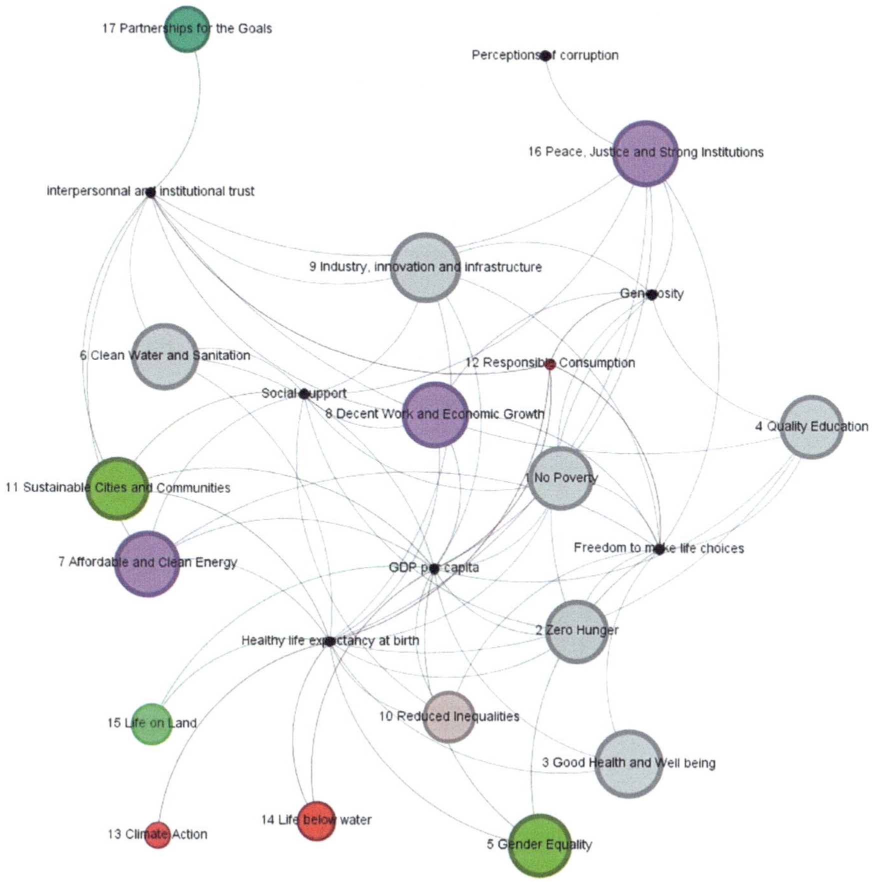

Fig. 2 Network of SDG and variables of happiness

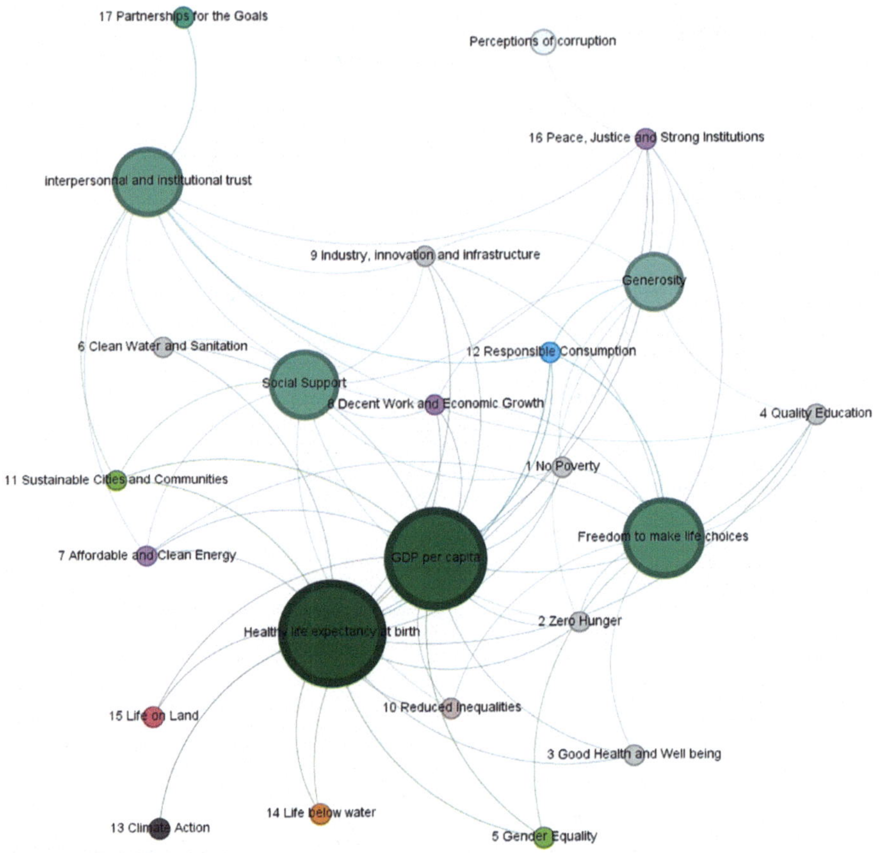

Fig. 3 Influence of SDG investments on happiness factors

3 Conclusion

As noted in the World Happiness Report (2023), the UN Sustainable Development Goals (SDGs) are also a vital component of the happiness agenda. From the network representations we illustrate the interdependencies and interconnectivity across the SDG and national Happiness variables. This points to the need for a complexity lens and systems thinking perspective when designing SDG intervention strategies. Policies designed must consider the holistic impact stemming from the influence across the network construct. In so doing, a conscious effort can be designed into policies to raise the happiness levels of a nation. This becomes Happiness by Design.

References

Araki, S. (2023). The societal determinants of happiness and unhappiness: Evidence from 152 Countries over 15 years. *Social Psychological and Personality Science, 1–13*, 1.

Badri, M. A., Alkhaili, M., Aldhaheri, H., Yang, G., Albahar, M., & Alrashdi, A. (2022). Exploring the reciprocal relationships between happiness and life satisfaction of working adults evidence from Abu Dhabi. *International Journal of Environmental Research and Public Health, 19*, 3575.

Barabasi, A.-L. (2016). *Network Science*. Cambridge University Press.

Boulton, J. G., Allen, P. M., Bowman, C. (2015). Embracing Complexity: Strategic Perspectives for an Age of Turbulence. Oxford University Press.

Capra, F. (2005). Complexity and Life Theory. *Culture Society, 22*, 33–44.

Cilliers, P. (1998). *Complexity and postmodernism: Understanding complex systems*. Routledge Publishing.

Coenen, J., Glass, L. M., & Sanderink, L. (2022). Two degrees and the SDGs: A network analysis of the interlinkages between transnational climate actions and the sustainable development goals. *Sustainability Science, 17*, 1489–1510.

Dawes, J. H. P. (2022). SDG interlinkage networks: Analysis, robustness, sensitivities, and hierarchies. *World Development, 149*, 1.

Easley, D., & Kleinberg, J. (2010). *Networks, Crowds and Markets: Reasoning about a highly connected world*. Cambridge University Press.

Fortier, F. (2020) Connecting the SDG dots through systems thinking. UN Staff College. https://www.unssc.org/sites/default/files/u3/systems_thinking_for_a2030.pdf

Gentili, P. L. (2021). Why is complexity science valuable for reaching the goals of the UN 2030 Agenda? *Rendiconti Lincei Scienze Fisiche e Naturali, 32*, 117–134.

Harvard (ND) https://www.hsph.harvard.edu/health-happiness/health-and-happiness-facts/

Helliwell, J. F., Layard, R., Sachs, J. D., & De Neve, J. E. (2020). World happiness report 2020. Sustainable Development Solutions Network.

Helliwell, J. F., Layard, R., Sachs, J. D., De Neve, J. E., Aknin, L. B., &Wang, S. (2021). World happiness report 2021. Sustainable Development Solutions Network.

Helliwell, J. F., Layard, R., Sachs, J. D., De Neve, J. E, Aknin, L. B., & Wang, S. (2022). World happiness report 2022. Sustainable Development Solutions Network.

Helliwell, J. F., Layard, R., Sachs, J. D., De Neve, J. E., Aknin, L. B., & Wang, S. (2023). World happiness report 2023. Sustainable Development Solutions Network.

Iriarte, L., & Musikanski, L. (2019). Bridging the gap between the sustainable development goals and happiness metrics. *International Journal of Community Well-Being, 1*, 115–135.

Laumann, F., von Kügelgen, J., Uehara, T. H. K., & Barahona, M. (2022). Complex interlinkages, key objectives, and nexuses among the sustainable development goals and climate change: A network analysis. *Lancet Planet Health, 2022*(6), e422–e430.

Le Blanc, D. (2015). Towards integration at last? The sustainable development goals as a network of targets. *Sustainable Development, 23*, 176–187.

Masys, A. J. (Ed.) (2021). Sensemaking for Security. Springer Publishing.

Masys, A. J. (2023). Impact Analysis of the War in Ukraine on Non-traditional Security: An Examination of the Emerging Risks to the Sustainable Development Goals. In TAdib Farhadi, Mark Grzegorzewski, Anthony J. Masys (Eds.) The Great Power Competition Volume 5 The Russian Invasion of Ukraine and Implications for the Central Region. Springer Publishing.

Medvedev, O. N., & Landhuis, C. E. (2018). Exploring constructs of well-being, happiness and quality of life. *Peer J, 6*, e4903.

Murthy, V. H. (2022). Confronting health worker burnout and well-being. *New England Journal of Medicine, 387*(7), 577–579.

Nemati, S., & Maralani, F. (2016). The relationship between life satisfaction and happiness: The mediating role of resiliency. *International Journal of Psychological Studies, 8*, 194–201.

Ottino, J. (2003). Complex systems. *AIChE Journal, 49*(2), 292–299.

Sachs, J. D. (2016). Chapter 4 Happiness and Sustainable Development: Concepts and Evidence. In John Helliwell, Richard Layard and Jeffrey Sachs (Eds.) World Happiness Report 2016.

Senge, P. (1990). *The Fifth Discipline: The Art and Practice of the Learning Organization.* Doubleday Currency.

Styhre, A. (2002). Non-linear change in organizations: Organization change management informed by complexity theory. *Leadership and Organization Development Journal, 23*(6), 343–351.

Sweeney, K., & Griffiths, F. (2002). *Complexity and healthcare: An introduction.* Radcliffe Medical press Ltd.

Theobald, T., & Cooper, C. (2012) Doing the Right Thing the Importance of Wellbeing in the Workplace. PALGRAVE MACMILLAN

UN DESA: https://www.un.org/development/desa/dspd/international-days/international-day-of happiness.html#:~:text=The%20General%20Assembly%20of%20the,importance%20o %20their%20recognition%20in

UN (2015) https://www.un.org/sustainabledevelopment/blog/2015/12/sustainable-development goals-kick-off-with-start-of-new-year/

UNDRR & UNU-EHS (2022). Understanding and managing cascading and systemic risks: lessonsfrom COVID-19. Geneva, UNDRR; Bonn, UNU-EHS

Urry, J. (2003). *Global Complexity.* Polity Press.

Weber, et al. (2021). (2020) Teaching sustainability as complex systems approach: A sustainable development goals workshop. *International Journal of Sustainability in Higher Education, 22*(8), 25–41.

WHO (2021) Health Promotion Glossary of Terms 2021. https://iris.who.int/bitstream/handle/10665/350161/9789240038349-eng.pdf?sequence=1

WHO (2022b) Achieving well-being a global framework for integrating well-being into public health utilizing a health promotion approach. https://www.who.int/publications/m/item/achieving-well-being

WHO (2022) https://www.who.int/news/item/02-03-2022-covid-19-pandemic-triggers25-increase-in-prevalence-of-anxiety-and-depression-worldwide

Zolli, A., & Healy, A. M. (2012). *Resilience: Why things bounce back.* Free Press.

Global Happiness and Humanitarian Assistance

3

Sara Spowart

Abstract

This chapter discusses and explores the significance and role of happiness in humanitarian assistance and global health work. It discusses the incorporation of happiness-based approaches and psychoeducation in well-being alongside humanitarian assistance interventions. The consideration of happiness should not be separate from humanitarian assistance, but part of trauma and intervention work. Depression is one of the greatest issues worldwide and currently causes the largest number of days of disability. Depression hinders health and development and is currently considered one of the most important health issues by the World Health Organization. It is also forecasted to continue to be the number one health issue worldwide into the foreseeable future. Psychoeducation and well-being strategies are effective ways to implement larger scale interventions to help decrease trauma, depression and acute stress due to humanitarian crisis and poverty.

Keywords

Humanitarian assistance • Psychoeducation • Global health • Vulnerable populations • Happiness

S. Spowart (✉)
University of South Florida, Tampa, FL, USA
e-mail: compassionbasedhappiness@gmail.com; sara.spowart@gmail.com

S. Spowart (ed.), *Global Happiness and Humanitarian Assistance*, Integrated Science 29, https://doi.org/10.1007/978-3-031-71789-5_3

1 Introduction

An estimated 250 million individuals suffer from anxiety disorders and 300 million experience depression worldwide. In addition to this, more than 80% of those suffering from anxiety and depression disorders live in low and middle-income countries. Moreover, those that live in low and middle-income countries are exposed to higher levels of hunger, food insecurity, social prejudice and marginalization, violence, trauma, stress, and poorer quality of life and psychosocial status. Generally, individuals living in poverty or extreme poverty have any underlying mental health disorders exasperated and are exposed to many severe stressors (Chikwira et al., 2022; Séverin, 2021; Wollburg, et al., 2023).

2 Mental Health and Global Health Security

According to the World Health Organization, mental health relates to mental and psychological well-being. Mental health is the most significant factor in happiness and subjective well-being. It refers to emotional, psychological, and social well-being. Mental health impacts our inner state of well-being and can negatively impact our physical health. It is significant for every stage of life, from childhood through adulthood into older age. Our state of mental health impacts how we have relationships, manage stress and make decisions (World Health Organization, 2020). At present, 94 countries or 48% of all World Health Organization Member States have worked on their policies for mental health in line with international and regional human rights standards. These countries have either newly created or updated laws to include mental health as a significant factor that should be considered by global health rights standards. At present and worldwide, the amount of public expenditure that goes to mental health is very small and inadequate in low and middle-income countries (World Health Organization, 2020).

Mental health is currently one of the most important global health and international development issues and has been recently added to the United Nations Sustainable Development Goals (SDGs). This is due to the evidence of how mental illness greatly contributes to overall disease burden. Mental health and economic development became more highlighted on the global health agenda through the WHO in 2010 with the 'Mental Health and Poverty Project.' This report highlights the association between mental health as a significant health factor and its connection to poverty. Implementing psychoeducation and poverty reduction in a joint venture is addressed as an effective global health security intervention (Mills, 2018). Also, the 130th session of the World Health Organization Executive Board adopted a declaration for a comprehensive response to the global burden of mental illness. The WHO estimates that major depression will be the greatest contributor to global disease burden by 2030. This means that it is an issue that only continues to rise at the moment. The impact of this level of depression and mental illness is incalculable; however, it is estimated it will comprise at least a 1/3 of the $47 trillion predicted global cost from non-communicable diseases by 2030 (Sachs et al., 2018; Sachs, 2017, 2018, 2019; Hock et al., 2012).

The United Nations World Health Organization reported that the percentage of people living with depression increased by 18% from 2005 to 2015. In 2017, the World Health Organization reported that over 800,000 people commit suicide every year. A large number of these are youth between the ages of 15–29 years (World Health Organization, 2017; Helliwell et al., 2017, 2013, 2018, 2020; Clark et al., 2017). According to the work of Santomauro et al. (2021), before 2020 mental illness was the leading cause of global health burden worldwide. Depression and anxiety were the main health issues within this disease framework. COVID worsened the disease burden already created by mental illness worldwide and increased the level of major depressive and anxiety disorders (Vahratian et al., 2021).

In 2019, the Global Burden of Diseases, Injuries and Risk Factors Study (GBD) demonstrated that depression and anxiety were the worst mental health issues worldwide and ranked in the top 25 health burden causes in 2019. It was found to be high across the whole lifespan, for male and females, and throughout many regions and countries (Santomauro et al, 2021). According to this study, there has been no reduction in worldwide prevalence and disease burden for anxiety or depression since 1990 and approximately 246 million suffer from major depressive disorder worldwide as of 2020 (Santomauro et al., 2021). Major depressive disorder and anxiety were among the top-ranking mental health and global health concerns before the COVID pandemic. Now these numbers have only worsened in prevalence and severity (Santomauro et al, 2021).

According to the American Medical Association, depression is the leading cause of disability worldwide (Helliwell et al., 2017, 2013, 2018, 2020; Clark et al., 2017). In many ways, depression is the consequence of low levels of happiness and has a significant, negative impact on poverty and development. Depression can express itself through loss of interest in things that used to bring joy, low levels of motivation, changes in appetite and sleep, difficulty concentrating, low levels of energy and lethargy, anger or irritability, and suicidal ideation. Depression can be the result of a sense of hopelessness and powerlessness. Individuals that are in a humanitarian crisis often experience both of these. There are effective treatments for depression. Some of these treatments include cognitive behavioral therapy, interpersonal mental health therapy, and medications such as antidepressants (Helliwell et al., 2017, 2013, 2018, 2020; Clark et al., 2017). Depression levels are highest among females in the African region; and rates of depression are highest in older adulthood, specifically from 55 to 74 years of age (Helliwell et al., 2017, 2013, 2018, 2020; Clark et al., 2017).

Yet, despite its importance for poverty reduction and development, the quantity of mental health workers is largely inadequate across the world. There are an estimated 72 mental health workers per 100,000 population in high-income countries and 1 mental health worker per 100,000 population in low-income countries. The global median number of mental health workers per 100,000 is 9 but there is major variation between low and high-income countries for access and type of treatment (World Health Organization, 2020; Helliwell et al., 2018). However, in both high and low-income countries, mental health treatment is inadequately provided. Furthermore, more than 80% of this public expenditure is directed towards funding mental hospitals, not to regular outpatient treatment. Mental health hospitals address the most acute, short-term mental health concerns and do not work in the community for prevention and treatment. A bulk of public health funding is directed toward mental hospitals. This is a reactive, high-cost approach that increases the chance of disability due to mental illness. It is inadequate for reducing mental health issues on a wider scale for a range of mental health conditions (World Health Organization, 2020; Helliwell et al., 2013, 2017, 2020, 2018).

Low-income populations are in general, more likely to experience trauma and Post-Traumatic Stress Syndrome (PTSD). They are also more likely to need microfinance intervention, health education and other types of humanitarian assistance and development support. Many of these populations are living with undiagnosed and untreated PTSD, and often experience discrimination, poverty, and handicaps such as chronic mental or physical illness. Individuals with severe mental illness almost universally have trauma exposure to one or multiple traumas. This trauma and trauma treatment is greatly underdiagnosed and untreated worldwide. Individuals exposed to trauma, often struggle with other issues such as poverty, depression, chronic medical conditions and substance use disorders. These populations are globally underserved and less likely to seek assistance after a traumatic event. Mindfulness, Cognitive Behavior Therapy, mental health first aid, psychoeducation with cognitive restructuring, and exposure therapy are useful interventions for trauma (Ruducha & Jadhav, 2018; Ortet et al., 2020; Kabat-Zinn, 2021; Mueser et al., 2009).

3 Psychoeducation and Humanitarian Assistance

The landscape of humanitarian assistance has changed in the last decades. In the past there was a focus on infectious disease, vaccinations and medical treatments. However, in the last couple decades there has been a shift towards non-communicable diseases such as heart disease, cancer, diabetes, addiction and contributing factors such as obesity, age, lifestyle and well-being. In the most recent years, there has been a shift from physical disease to the importance of mental health issues. Although it is not sufficiently documented to this day, it is estimated that the worst levels and highest prevalence of mental illness, (specifically anxiety and depression disorders) exist in low and middle-income countries.

These regions generally have poor mental health literacy, knowledge, access and availability of treatment (World Health Organization, 2021, 2018a, 2018b).

Given this, psychoeducation is a supportive approach with the potential to reduce mental illness and even severe mental illness symptoms. Psychoeducation is a systematic, structured, didactic approach to addressing mental illness and intervention tools. Psychoeducation helps families and patients to better understand mental health and how to address it (Marquez & Main, 2021; Martinez, 2015; Srivastava & Panday, 2016). According to Jones et al. (2018a, 2018b), psychoeducation can provide an effective approach for self-management of health issues (McRae & Gross, 2020). Fifteen studies were reviewed in an investigation conducted by Jones, Stone et al. (2018) and it was found that psychoeducational interventions can prevent and reduce depression as both a first-line direct or supportive tool (Jones et al., 2018a, 2018b; Srivastava & Panday, 2016).

There are multiple forms of psychoeducation. Some of these include what are termed the Information, Skill Training, Supportive and Comprehensive Models. The Information Model works to provide families with information on psychiatric illness and its management. It is intended to improve a family's awareness regarding an illness and its management. The Skill Training Model is aimed at increasing certain behaviors so that family members and individuals can better manage and understand a mental health condition. The Supportive Model uses support groups to improve the ability of families and individuals to manage a mental health condition. The Comprehensive model or combination approach applies information, skill training and the supportive model to address a mental health phenomenon. It consists of information and knowledge regarding the condition, support groups, and lastly individual sessions with a mental health professional regarding the phenomenon (Srivastava & Panday, 2016).

4 The Value of Combined Humanitarian Assistance and Psychoeducation Interventions

Low-income populations have higher rates of depression and trauma and need additional support aside from economic empowerment to improve their health, overall circumstances and well-being (Asnaani et al., 2020; Alesane, 2023; Bika et al., 2022). Trauma here refers to exposure to a traumatic or triggering event. This may be exposure to an actual or threatened death, serious injury, abuse, violence, or sexual violence. Trauma refers to events that cause threats to one's survival or physical existence and is commonly experienced in humanitarian assistance situations. It can refer to not only trauma from events that have occurred to individuals, but also to traumatic events such as violence or death to others of familial connection (Whitworth, 2016).

Trauma psychoeducation is increasingly popular and can help someone understand how the trauma they experienced can impact their functioning and how to manage those impacts. Trauma psychoeducation can be used before or after exposure to a traumatic event. Important goals of trauma-focused psychoeducation include an increased understanding of common trauma reactions, and skills and knowledge to manage those reactions. Psychoeducation on trauma is more impactful when resilience and recovery is emphasized, not only painful trauma symptoms. This education should help participants feel empowered, more resilient and understand that their trauma experience is connected to their trauma reactions (Kim-Prieto et al., 2005; Klussman et al., 2022; Korkmaz, 2021; Whitworth, 2016).

Certain components make psychoeducation in humanitarian assistance situations more effective. This includes an emphasis on resilience, adaptation, self-care, self-compassion, and building and maintaining supportive relationships. Individuals that have experienced threats, sexual assault, neglect and other types of abuse, often struggle to form supportive relationships. Positive, supportive, interpersonal relationships can help lessen the impact of trauma reactions, and provide greater connection and safety. Psychoeducation can also integrate practical tools like mindfulness, relaxation training, yoga, emotional support animals, music therapy and other forms of support (Kim-Prieto et al., 2005; Klussman et al., 2022; Korkmaz, 2021; Mehrabi et al., 2017; Whitworth, 2016). Groups that provide health education, financial or literacy support, and other forms of humanitarian assistance can integrate psychoeducation into their curriculum (Lorenzetti et al., 2017; *The Association des Femmes du Mali pour la Solidarite el le Developpement*, personal communication, July 15, 2023; *Espoir des Femmes et des Enfants du Mali* (EFEM), personal communication, July 15, 2023).

5 Challenges in Implementing Sustainable Psychoeducation Programs for At-Need Groups

There can be many challenges in implementing psychoeducation programs for at-need groups. Some of these challenges include a lack of knowledge regarding psychoeducation, social stigma, and awareness of how it will strengthen humanitarian assistance development initiatives.

Depression with its corresponding hopelessness, decreased motivation, and energy, directly impacts development levels in at-need populations. Populations living in absolute poverty suffer from higher levels of mental illness and conditions such as depression. Therefore, happiness-based mindfulness programs and interventions are useful for development, progress, and progression. Communities and populations are not able to reach their full potential for development when plagued by severe depression and trauma symptoms.Query

"Yes, we struggle with hunger and eating only 1–2 times a day and just millet. But really the biggest problem is feeling hopelessness, darkness, and that nothing will change. The biggest problem is depression. We go through the landfill here to survive, but the worst thing is feeling there is no hope." (Freedom From Hunger, Espoir des Femmes et des Enfants du Mali (EFEM, & The Association des Femmes

du Mali pour la Solidarite et le Developpement, verbal communication with focus group participants of a Mali hunger program, 2009 & 2023).

6 Important Elements of Psychoeducation and Humanitarian Assistance for At-Need Populations and Groups

There are effective types of psychoeducation for humanitarian assistance programs. Topics that address the impact of stress, trauma, abuse and relationships can positively impact participants. Other supportive subjects include education on self-care, grounding exercises, the window of distress tolerance, triggers and healthy versus unhealthy relationships (Hershler, 2021). Another effective intervention was created by author, Sara Spowart PhD, LMFT, the Happiness-Based Mindfulness Program (HBMP). This is a psychoeducation program with concrete tangible tools. There are four formats. These include a Brief Trauma-Focused format, a Youth-Focused format, a 6-Week version, as well as the intensive, in-depth 12-Week version. Each session is comprised of clearly described curriculum and criteria, with exercises that can be easily adapted and replicable in many situations, cultures, and languages (Spowart, 2024).

7 The Happiness-Based Mindfulness Program

The Happiness-Based Mindfulness Program and the Brief Trauma-Focused format are structured psychoeducation programs that are meant to help provide support for individuals regardless of the circumstances they are in. It incorporates certain aspects of happiness and mindfulness that the author has identified in her career and research that are most positively impactful for improving well-being. The program can be adapted to fit crises, long-term development circumstances, violence, and long-term chronic poverty circumstances. It can be adapted in a long or short format for either an individual or group psychoeducational intervention. The author has created a Brief Trauma-Focused version that can be potentially applied to humanitarian assistance interventions. It can be found in the appendix section of this chapter (Spowart, 2022, 2024).

Core components of the Happiness-Based Mindfulness Program and the Brief Trauma-Focused HBMP include the emotion chart that contains the Red, Green and Blue Zones. This chart can be viewed in the Appendix section, under Appendix A. The Red Zone refers to an area that contains destructive emotions, the Green Zone are relief emotions and the Blue Zones are lightening and uplifting emotions. Creating awareness and identifying where you are in the chart zones helps no matter where you are existing in the spectrum of emotions. This program includes weekly meetings and meditation recordings to help with more positive thinking and letting go of trauma and pain. Additional components of both programs include simplified and adapted Rational Emotive Behavior Therapy (REBT) exercises. These exercises work to provide straightforward tools to adjust and reframe negative and painful beliefs and rework to more empowering and uplifting perspectives. The adapted REBT exercise can be found in Appendix B of this chapter (Spowart, 2022, 2024).

Another unique component of both the Happiness-Based Mindfulness Program and the Brief Trauma-Focused HBMP is the practice with the Identity Circle and the Trapped Cycles Exercise, created by author Sara Spowart, PhD. The Identity Circle is an analysis exercise to help understand different levels of self and who is the authentic self within this. A major component of unhappiness or happiness is the way we define ourselves and others, and labels we place on ourselves. However, a lot of times there has not been a clear investigation for our perceived identity and attachment we have to our identity structure that may shift with life events and tragedies. We may define ourselves in negative ways, or not know how to define ourselves after trauma and crisis occurs. Therefore, this activity is an opportunity to define ourselves in positive ways that promote empowerment and resilience. The "Identity Circle" can be found in Appendix C at the end of this chapter (Spowart, 2022, 2024). The Trapped Cycles exercise can be found in Appendix D at the end of this chapter. It helps individuals assess if they are trapped in any repeating patterns in their lives, what they are stuck in, and ways to get out of repeating, harmful cycles in an easy-to-understand, clear, and visualized way (Spowart, 2022, 2024).

Two other important tools are the Compassion-Based Resiliency Chart and the Nervous System, Safety & Rest Exercise. These tools are used for the Brief Trauma-Focused HBMP. The Compassion-Based Resiliency Chart incorporates aspects of mindfulness and compassion to help participants increase levels of well-being. It can be found in Appendix E at the end of this chapter. The Nervous System, Safety & Rest Exercise is used to help participants reduce their levels of stress, trauma, and negative emotion by physiologically calming the body and then mind. It can be found in Appendix F at the end of this chapter.

8 Conclusion

This chapter provides an overview of the relevance of psychoeducation initiatives for low-income, at-need populations. It also highlights the intersection of positive mental health and humanitarian assistance. Humanitarian assistance interventions that include happiness and psychoeducation initiatives are likely much more effective and positively impactful for creating sustainable change. Interventions that apply the component of happiness along with humanitarian assistance are needed to improve the well-being of the world's most vulnerable populations. The principles of the Happiness-Based Mindfulness Program and Brief Trauma-Focused HBMP demonstrate that happiness can be taught and learned through concrete, psychoeducational tools and interventions. There are tangible tools to teach and learn to increase your happiness, and these tools are simple, straightforward, and easy to learn on your own and in a group and to integrate into your life even after the program. The author of this chapter has applied these tools for thousands of client sessions with significant positive outcomes and results. Further practice, application, and research are needed for greater understanding and larger widescale application for humanitarian assistance situations.

Acknowledgements I would like to acknowledge The Association des Femmes du Mali pour la Solidarite el le Developpement (AFMSD), PenPath Volunteers, The Gambia Children's Fund, The Hanang Orphan and Street Children Project, Espoir des Femmes et des Enfants du Mali (EFEM) and Compassion-Based Happiness, LLC for their invaluable contributions to this chapter.

Conflict of interest The authors declare no conflict of interest.

Thanks Thank you to *Compassion-Based Happiness*, LLC, *PenPath Volunteers, The Gambia Children's Fund, The Hanang Orphan and Street Children Project, Espoir des Femmes et des Enfants du Mali* (EFEM) and *The Association des Femmes du Mali pour la Solidarite et le Developpement* for your invaluable contributions to this chapter.

Appendices

Appendix A

Emotion Chart

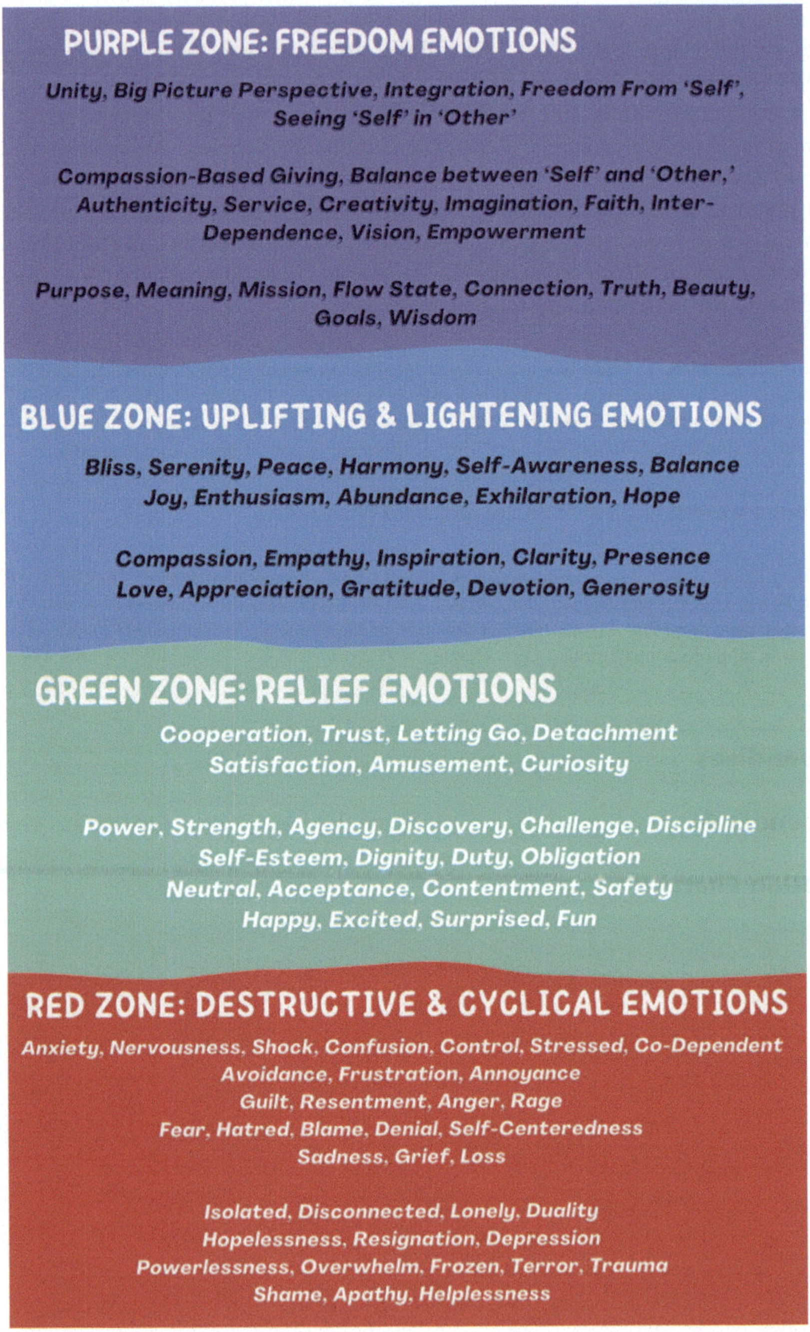
PURPLE ZONE: FREEDOM EMOTIONS
Unity, Big Picture Perspective, Integration, Freedom From 'Self', Seeing 'Self' in 'Other'
Compassion-Based Giving, Balance between 'Self' and 'Other,' Authenticity, Service, Creativity, Imagination, Faith, Inter-Dependence, Vision, Empowerment
Purpose, Meaning, Mission, Flow State, Connection, Truth, Beauty, Goals, Wisdom
BLUE ZONE: UPLIFTING & LIGHTENING EMOTIONS
Bliss, Serenity, Peace, Harmony, Self-Awareness, Balance
Joy, Enthusiasm, Abundance, Exhilaration, Hope
Compassion, Empathy, Inspiration, Clarity, Presence
Love, Appreciation, Gratitude, Devotion, Generosity
GREEN ZONE: RELIEF EMOTIONS
Cooperation, Trust, Letting Go, Detachment
Satisfaction, Amusement, Curiosity
Power, Strength, Agency, Discovery, Challenge, Discipline
Self-Esteem, Dignity, Duty, Obligation
Neutral, Acceptance, Contentment, Safety
Happy, Excited, Surprised, Fun
RED ZONE: DESTRUCTIVE & CYCLICAL EMOTIONS
Anxiety, Nervousness, Shock, Confusion, Control, Stressed, Co-Dependent
Avoidance, Frustration, Annoyance
Guilt, Resentment, Anger, Rage
Fear, Hatred, Blame, Denial, Self-Centeredness
Sadness, Grief, Loss
Isolated, Disconnected, Lonely, Duality
Hopelessness, Resignation, Depression
Powerlessness, Overwhelm, Frozen, Terror, Trauma
Shame, Apathy, Helplessness

Appendix B: Adapted REBT

Adapted Rational Emotive Behavior Therapy (REBT) Exercise Example:

Negative Identified Belief:

- There's no reason to be happy

  What is the benefit of this negative identified belief?

- I get more attention from my family and others when i feel sad

  What is the harm of this negative identified belief?
  Feeling Bad, not Helping Mood or Wanting to Stay Sober

3 Positive Alternatives to Identified Belief:

(a) There is at least one reason to be happy.
(b) Eventually there could be a reason to be happy.
(c) I am mostly just hurting myself with this belief.

Appendix C: Identity Circle

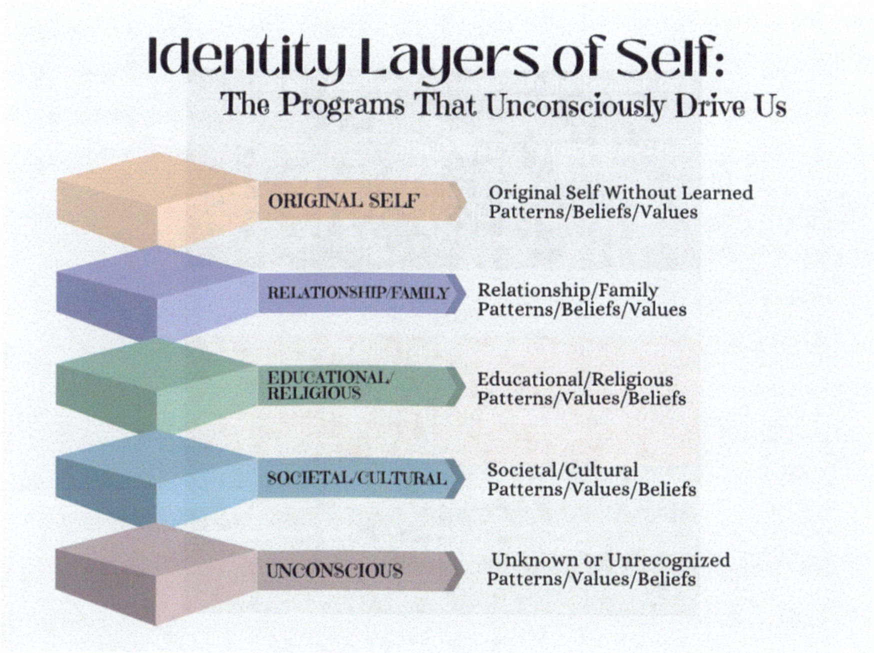

Appendix D: Trapped Cycles

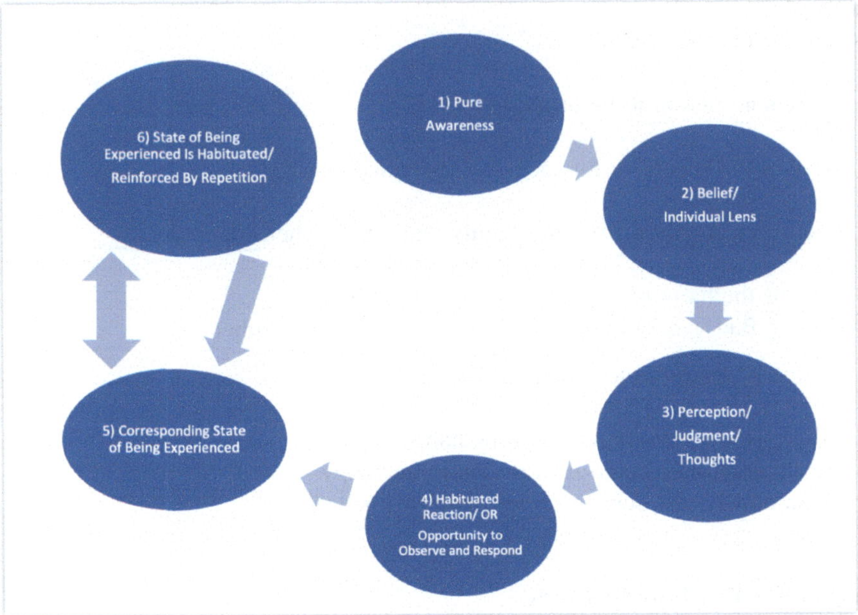

Appendix E: Compassion-Based Resiliency Chart

Full, Unconditional Compassion to Self and Others
Full Compassion to Self and Others
Partial Compassion to Self and Others
Neutral on Compassion to Self and Others
Partial Negative Judgement of Self and Others
Full Negative Judgement of Self and Others
Don't Understand or Know What This Means
Unconscious Reactions, Habits and Patterns

Appendix F: The Nervous System, Safety & Rest Exercise

- Close your eyes and sit in a comfortable position, and maybe with your feet on the floor
- Take a deep breath in through your nose and out through your mouth
- Take another deep breath in through your nose and out through your mouth
- Take one more deep breath in through your nose and out through your mouth
- And as I Count Down from 5 to 1, Feeling More and More Relaxed, Calm and at Peace
- 5–4 Feeling More Relaxed
- 4–3
- 3–2 Calmer and Calmer
- 2–1 Feeling Calm, Relaxed and at Peace
- Imagine that You Are Sitting Near a Grassy Green Field and Peaceful Forest
- Breath in Peace and Calm
- Breath Out the Feeling of Support and Safety
- Notice the Breath in and Out and the Flow of the Air
- Now, Imagine You Are Standing up and then Are Walking Towards the Forest
- As You Walk Towards the Forest, You Feel More and More Supported, Calm and at Peace
- Deep Breath in and Out, Allowing Yourself in This Moment to Be Safe and Supported
- Breathing in Support and Compassion
- Breathing Out Support and Compassion
- Then imagine that you are wearing a back-pack full of rocks, and these rocks are everything and anything that is weighing you down, causing you trauma, stress, pain and fear
- You walk over to a lake in the forest, and this lake dissolves any and all the rocks in your backpack
- One by one throwing these rocks into the lake, and they melt and dissolve away
- 3
- 2
- And 1
- These rocks melt and dissolve away completely
- And throwing your backpack into the lake now, and it dissolves away completely
- And you feel lighter and lighter, more and more at peace and at ease
- Deep breath in and out,
- Imagining yourself sitting in this forest by the lake
- *And you are filled with rest*
- *Your head, neck and shoulders…in this moment, it is safe to rest*

- *Your arms and hands ….in this moment, it is safe to rest*
- *Your torso, heart, chest, and stomach…rest*
- *Your back, hips, legs and feet…all rest*
- *And you breath in a feeling of rest and relaxation, and breath out*
- *Knowing that in this moment, it is safe to rest, relax and experience some peace*
- …

Appendix G: Brief Trauma-Focused HBMP

(Adapted for Use in Humanitarian Assistance Initiatives)

Brief Trauma-Focused HBMP

Created by Sara Spowart, LMFT, PhD
Session 1: Helpless and Powerless

When major life changes, stressors or traumas occur, we can feel lost, confused, helpless and powerless. Everything we thought we knew can be destroyed or in chaos. It can seem impossible to know what to trust or count on, or how to make sense of the tragedies, extreme stress and suffering.

In this session we work on and explore understanding the Emotion Chart Exercise and the Red, Green and Blue zones of this chart. We also explore discussion and reflection on the emotions we are currently experiencing and how to go from feelings of helplessness and powerlessness into greater strength, resilience and hope. This exercise is also continued in Session 2.

In addition to this, we work on the topic of compassion in this session through the Compassion-Based Resiliency Exercise. Compassion here referring to a sense of kindness and love, combined with insight and understanding of life situation. This compassion refers not only to compassion for ourselves but for others and our life situations. Our levels of compassion help impact our resiliency, recovery, mindset and perspective. They can bring ease to challenging circumstances and uplift us in times of crisis.

Lastly in session 1, there is the Nervous System, Safety and Rest Exercise. This is a relaxation, deep breathing, meditation exercise meant to help reduce nervous system distress. In times of crisis, extreme stress and trauma, exercises that help calm the nervous system can be deeply beneficial and help to reset our systems. If our nervous is on overdrive from traumatic stress, it greatly heightens the chances of physical and mental illness. It also makes it much more challenging to manage everyday stressors and life functioning. This exercise is continued also in Session 2.

First Exercise:
(1) The Emotion Chart Exercise (Approximately 15 min):
Emotion Chart

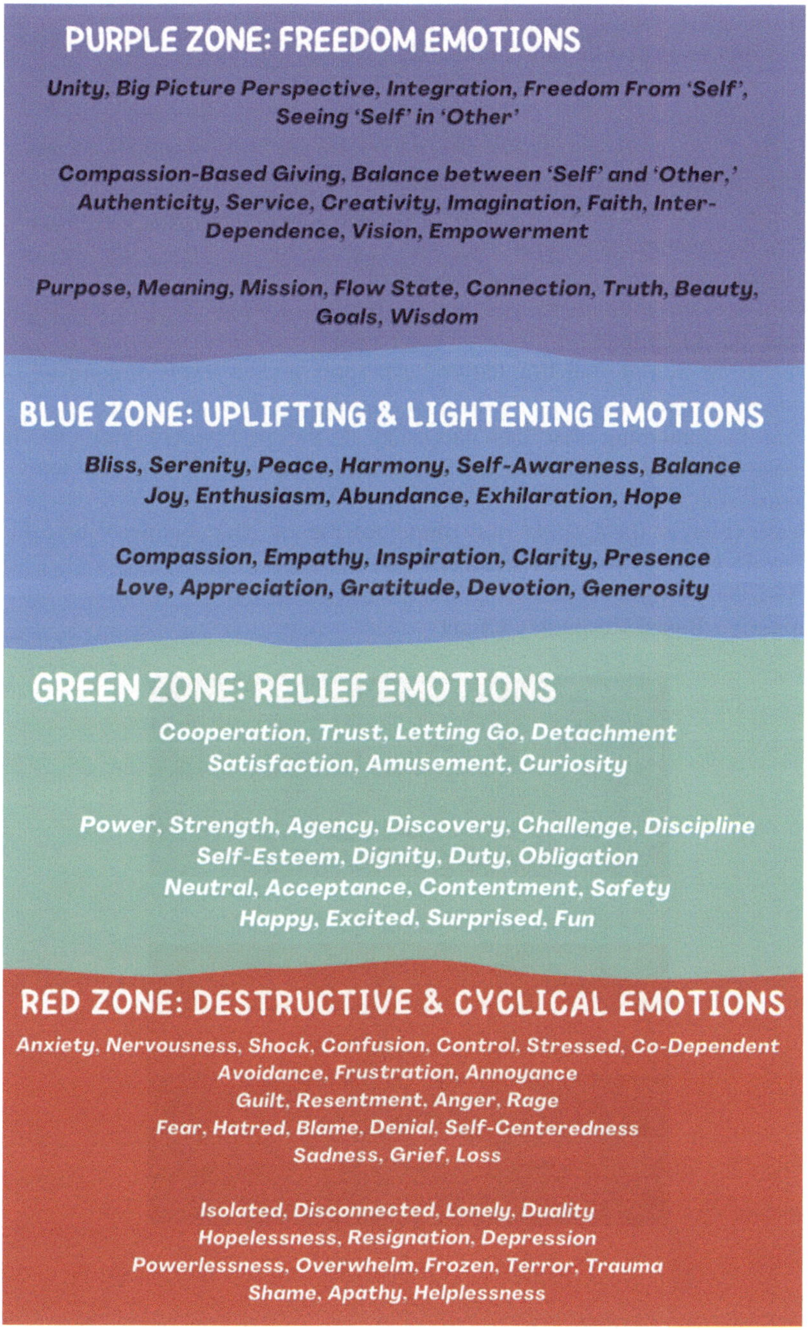

Reflection and Discussion Questions:

a. Where have you been in the chart today or right now…the *Red*, *Green* and/or *Blue Zones*?
b. How much are you in these different zones?
c. What emotions do you most frequently experience?

Second Exercise:

(2) The Compassion-Based Resiliency Exercise (Approximately 30–45 min):

Reflection and Discussion Questions:

a. What does *compassion* mean for you?
b. b. What does *compassion for others* mean?
c. When are some moments you have experienced some level of compassion? What did it feel like?
d. What is an area of your life that you can apply greater levels of compassion to yourself or others currently? How can you apply this compassion?
e. What is something that has happened in the past where you can apply greater levels of compassion for yourself or others? How can you apply this compassion?
f. Please refer to the Compassion-Based Resiliency chart below. Where in the chart do you feel you are recently?

Compassion-Based Resiliency Chart

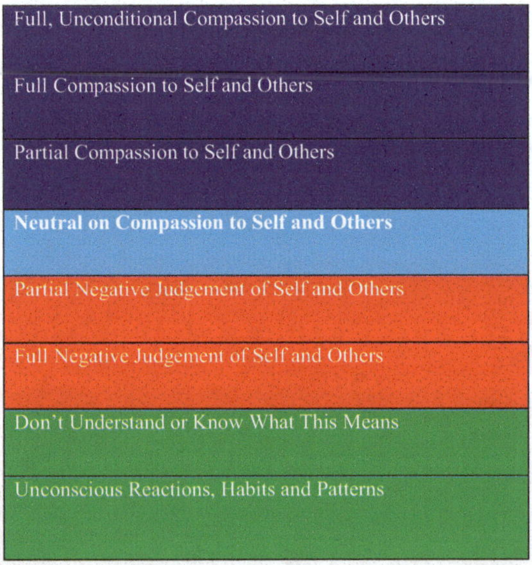

Third Exercise:
(3) the Nervous System, Safety & Rest Exercise (Approximately 15 min):

- Close your eyes and sit in a comfortable position, and maybe with your feet on the floor
- Take a deep breath in through your nose and out through your mouth
- Take another deep breath in through your nose and out through your mouth
- Take one more deep breath in through your nose and out through your mouth
- And as i count down from 5 to 1, feeling more and more relaxed, calm and at peace
- 5–4 Feeling more relaxed
- 4–3
- 3–2 Calmer and calmer
- 2–1 Feeling calm, relaxed and at peace
- Imagine that you are sitting near a grassy green field and peaceful forest
- Breath in peace and calm
- Breath out the feeling of support and safety
- Notice the breath in and out and the flow of the air
- Now, imagine you are standing up and then are walking towards the forest
- As you walk towards the forest, you feel more and more supported, calm and at peace
- Deep breath in and out, allowing yourself in this moment to be safe and supported
- Breathing in support and compassion
- Breathing out support and compassion
- Then imagine that you are wearing a back-pack full of rocks, and these rocks are everything and anything that is weighing you down, causing you trauma, stress, pain and fear
- You walk over to a lake in the forest, and this lake dissolves any and all the rocks in your backpack
- One by one throwing these rocks into the lake, and they melt and dissolve away
- 3
- 2
- And 1
- These rocks melt and dissolve away completely
- And throwing your backpack into the lake now, and it dissolves away completely
- And you feel lighter and lighter, more and more at peace and at ease
- Deep breath in and out,
- Imagining yourself sitting in this forest by the lake
- And you are filled with rest

- Your head, neck and shoulders…in this moment, it is safe to rest
- Your arms and hands ….in this moment, it is safe to rest
- Your torso, heart, chest, and stomach…rest
- Your back, hips, legs and feet…all rest
- And you breath in a feeling of rest and relaxation, and breath out
- Knowing that in this moment, it is safe to rest, relax and experience some peace
- …

Session 2: Positive, Resilient Self

When an individual or group experiences trauma, severe stress, violence, powerlessness, hopelessness, or other things similar to this…it is not unusual to struggle with self-worth and self-confidence. Survivors of trauma or abuse often suffer from lower self-esteem, and negative, depressive thought patterns and blame themselves for what they have experienced. This can be a way to cope with and try to make sense of things that are beyond our understanding. However, ultimately, negativity towards the self, negative thought patterns or beliefs, and staying in the victim or weakened mindset, only makes things worse in the end.

Our ability to foster and support a positive, resilient self is essential for strengthening ourselves to handle difficult, or traumatic life circumstances. No matter what the situation is, we can shift our mindset or perspective to help us become stronger and more empowered. The exercises covered in this session include the Emotion Chart Exercise, The Positive Identity Circle Exercise and The Nervous System, Safety & Rest Exercise.

The Emotion Chart Exercise is meant to help foster an awareness and comprehension for what emotions you are experiencing and the main zones you are living in, if these are the red, green or blue zones or some combination.

The Positive Identity Circle Exercise is meant to help identity and reflect on what beliefs or thoughts you hold about yourself, your community and situation. It is an opportunity to reflect on how you view yourself, your community and environment and any beliefs you'd like to keep or change to better empower yourself. A positive identity is very powerful for resiliency and optimism in your own strengths and abilities, and ability to manage traumatic and high stress situations. The way we view ourselves, others and our community are powerful for how we navigate unknown or traumatic life circumstances and getting beyond them.

The Nervous System, Safety & Rest Exercise is the last exercise in this session and is also significant in its ability to foster and support greater inner strength, resiliency and healing. Trauma and severe stress due to humanitarian situations and disasters can be very hard on the nervous system and our daily living. It can negatively impact our thinking, mindset, ability to rebuild or navigate challenging circumstances, thrive, be successful and heal. By calming the nervous system, we can experience greater restoration, healing and even post-traumatic growth after severely stressful and painful life situations. It is recommended to do this exercise or a similar one every day to help calm the mind, body and nervous system, no matter what the circumstances may be.

First Exercise:
(1) Emotion Chart Exercise (Approximately 15 min):
Emotion Chart

PURPLE ZONE: FREEDOM EMOTIONS

Unity, Big Picture Perspective, Integration, Freedom From 'Self', Seeing 'Self' in 'Other'

Compassion-Based Giving, Balance between 'Self' and 'Other,' Authenticity, Service, Creativity, Imagination, Faith, Inter-Dependence, Vision, Empowerment

Purpose, Meaning, Mission, Flow State, Connection, Truth, Beauty, Goals, Wisdom

BLUE ZONE: UPLIFTING & LIGHTENING EMOTIONS

Bliss, Serenity, Peace, Harmony, Self-Awareness, Balance
Joy, Enthusiasm, Abundance, Exhilaration, Hope

Compassion, Empathy, Inspiration, Clarity, Presence
Love, Appreciation, Gratitude, Devotion, Generosity

GREEN ZONE: RELIEF EMOTIONS

Cooperation, Trust, Letting Go, Detachment
Satisfaction, Amusement, Curiosity

Power, Strength, Agency, Discovery, Challenge, Discipline
Self-Esteem, Dignity, Duty, Obligation
Neutral, Acceptance, Contentment, Safety
Happy, Excited, Surprised, Fun

RED ZONE: DESTRUCTIVE & CYCLICAL EMOTIONS

Anxiety, Nervousness, Shock, Confusion, Control, Stressed, Co-Dependent
Avoidance, Frustration, Annoyance
Guilt, Resentment, Anger, Rage
Fear, Hatred, Blame, Denial, Self-Centeredness
Sadness, Grief, Loss

Isolated, Disconnected, Lonely, Duality
Hopelessness, Resignation, Depression
Powerlessness, Overwhelm, Frozen, Terror, Trauma
Shame, Apathy, Helplessness

Reflection and Discussion Questions:

a. Where have you been in the chart today or right now…the *Red*, *Green* and/or *Blue Zones*?
b. How much are you in these different zones?
c. What is a "Blue or Green Zone" emotion you'd like to experience more of? How can you do 5 minutes a day of something small to bring this experience into your life?

Second Exercise:

(2) ***The Positive Identity Circle Exercise*** *(approximately 20 min)***:**

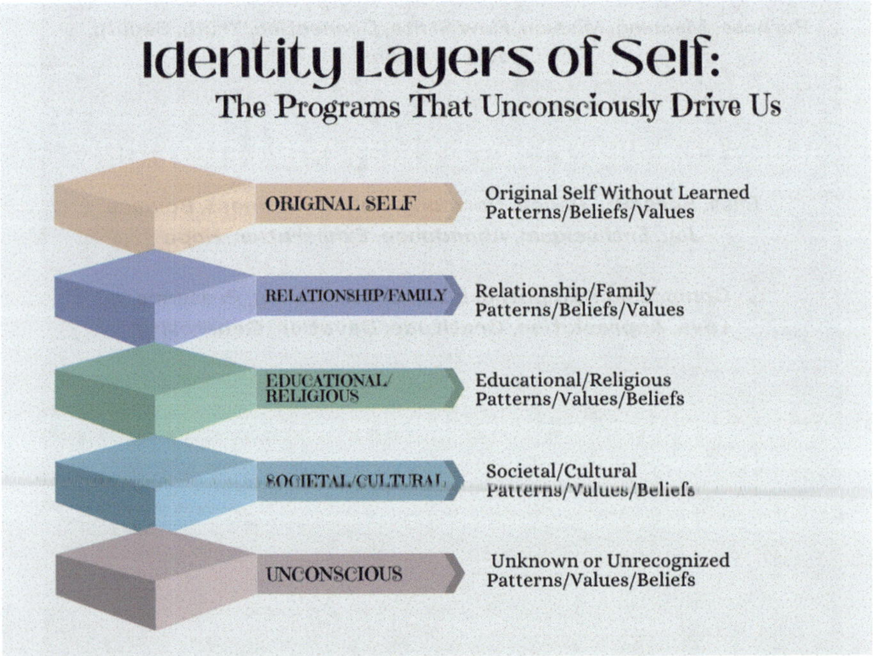

Reflection and Discussion Questions:

a. What are some patterns, values, or beliefs you hold about yourself that are positive?
b. What are some patterns, values or beliefs you hold about your family and close friends that are positive?
c. What are some patterns, values or beliefs you hold about your community that are positive?
d. Are there any patterns, values or beliefs you would like to have and add to your life that are positive?

Third Exercise:

(3) the Nervous System, Safety & Rest Exercise (Approximately 15 min):

Close Your Eyes and Sit in a Comfortable Position, and Maybe with Your Feet on the Floor

- Take a deep breath in through your nose and out through your mouth
- Take another deep breath in through your nose and out through your mouth
- Take one more deep breath in through your nose and out through your mouth
- And as i count down from 5 to 1, feeling more and more relaxed, calm and at peace
- 5–4 Feeling more relaxed
- 4–3
- 3–2 Calmer and calmer
- 2–1 Feeling calm, relaxed and at peace
- Imagine that you are sitting near a grassy green field and peaceful forest
- Breath in peace and calm
- Breath out the feeling of support and safety
- Notice the breath in and out and the flow of the air
- Now, imagine you are standing up and then are walking towards the forest
- As you walk towards the forest, you feel more and more supported, calm and at peace
- Deep breath in and out, allowing yourself in this moment to be safe and supported
- Breathing in support and compassion
- Breathing out support and compassion
- Then imagine that you are wearing a back-pack full of rocks, and these rocks are everything and anything that is weighing you down, causing you trauma, stress, pain and fear
- You walk over to a lake in the forest, and this lake dissolves any and all the rocks in your backpack
- One by one throwing these rocks into the lake, and they melt and dissolve away
- 3
- 2
- And 1
- These rocks melt and dissolve away completely
- And throwing your backpack into the lake now, and it dissolves away completely
- And you feel lighter and lighter, more and more at peace and at ease
- Deep breath in and out,
- Imagining yourself sitting in this forest by the lake
- And you are filled with rest

- Your head, neck and shoulders…in this moment, it is safe to rest
- Your arms and hands ….in this moment, it is safe to rest
- Your torso, heart, chest, and stomach…rest
- Your back, hips, legs and feet…all rest
- And you breath in a feeling of rest and relaxation, and breath out
- Knowing that in this moment, it is safe to rest, relax and experience some peace
- …

Session 3: Feeling Better

In this session, we look at our innate ability and the application of certain practices that can help bring greater freedom from suffering. There is a balance between validating and honoring our experiences and being free of their pain so we can thrive and somehow improve our situations. Part of overcoming suffering from traumatic life events or chronic toxic stress is to honor and validate what you have experienced and have compassion for yourself and your suffering. Even if what you experienced is considered 'normal' in your community, family, or society, it doesn't mean it didn't have a negative, painful impact. It doesn't mean things weren't done that were wrong or extremely harmful. However, normalizing or ignoring that pain and the experiences unfortunately will not make it go away. It can create harmful coping mechanisms or patterns that do not help you thrive and overcome and create issues like panic, severe anxiety, trauma symptoms, depression, hopelessness, and even suicidal ideation. However, if we become extremely focused on our pain and suffering and what we have experienced, and it even becomes part of our identity, that is also problematic. There is a balance and middle way to manage extreme suffering or trauma so it does not consume or define you or your life in the long term. The things that have happened in your life, the experiences you've had, and your current life situation doesn't have to be the end of your story or your identity. We can find a way to turn it into motivation for change, rebuilding, and growth.

In this session, we work on three exercises. The first is the Honor Your Suffering Exercise. In this, we work to validate and honor what we, others, or our community have experienced that has created trauma and great pain. The goal is not to become stuck in the pain, but rather to honor and acknowledge it for the power it has and our own unique experience of it. Then to apply compassion to the pain and ourselves. The second exercise in this session is the Adapted Rational Emotive Behavior Therapy (REBT) Exercise. This is an opportunity to learn a tangible skill to help transform negative thoughts, feelings, or beliefs into alternative, positive ones. The goal of this exercise is to provide information on a tangible skill that can be applied daily even after the session is done. The more you practice this activity, the more it becomes part of your everyday mindset and will help you manage stress, negative emotions, and future events. The third exercise is the Blue Zone Emotion Chart Exercise. This is adapted from the Emotion Chart Exercise conducted in the first and second sessions. The goal of this activity is to cultivate a greater focus on positive, 'blue zone' emotions and bring greater awareness to these emotions. By practicing noticing when you are having those emotions, and intentionally trying to create moments where you feel blue-zone emotions, you create more neuropathways in the brain that allow for more blue-zone thoughts and feelings. You also start to intentionally create more goodness in your life, even if it's just a small shift every day, or 1% happier every day or every week. Over time this adds up when we intentionally try to focus on experiencing a few moments in the Blue Zone.

First Exercise:

1 Honor Your Suffering Exercise (Approximately 20 min):

d. Please list at least 5 things that are upsetting you or 5 emotions you are struggling with such as guilt, anxiety, helplessness, powerlessness, overwhelm, sadness, fear, depression, stress, or shame.
e. Please discuss or write for 10 minutes on at least one of these 5 things
f. Then please reflect on compassion for these five things

Second Exercise:

2 Adapted Rational Emotive Behavior Therapy (REBT) Exercise (Approximately 20 min):

g. Please reflect on a negative thought or belief you have
h. Please discuss or write how this negative thought or belief may benefit you (usually it is a protective reason)
i. Please discuss or write how this negative thought or belief may harm you (usually it worsens life situation or negative emotions and puts you more in the 'Red Zone')
j. Please discuss or write at least 3 positive alternatives to this negative thought or belief

(1) Negative Identified Belief:

What is the Benefit of This Negative Identified Belief?

What is the Harm of This Negative Identified Belief?

3 Positive Alternatives to Identified Belief:

(a)
(B)
(C)

Third Exercise:
C. *Blue Zone Emotion Chart Exercise* *(approximately 10 min)***:**

k. Please look at the Blue Zone area of the chart below.
l. Are there any moments you experienced in the blue zone, even if it was 1 minute or less recently?
m. What blue zone emotion did you experience and why?
n. Can you try to create more blue zone emotions every day? If yes, which emotion would you like to try to focus on?

Uplifting and Lightening Emotions
Serenity, Peace, Harmony, Self-Awareness, Balance
Joy, Enthusiasm, Abundance, Exhilaration
Compassion, Empathy, Inspiration, Clarity, Presence
Love, Appreciation, Gratitude, Devotion, Generosity

Resources for the Sessions:

A. Emotion Chart

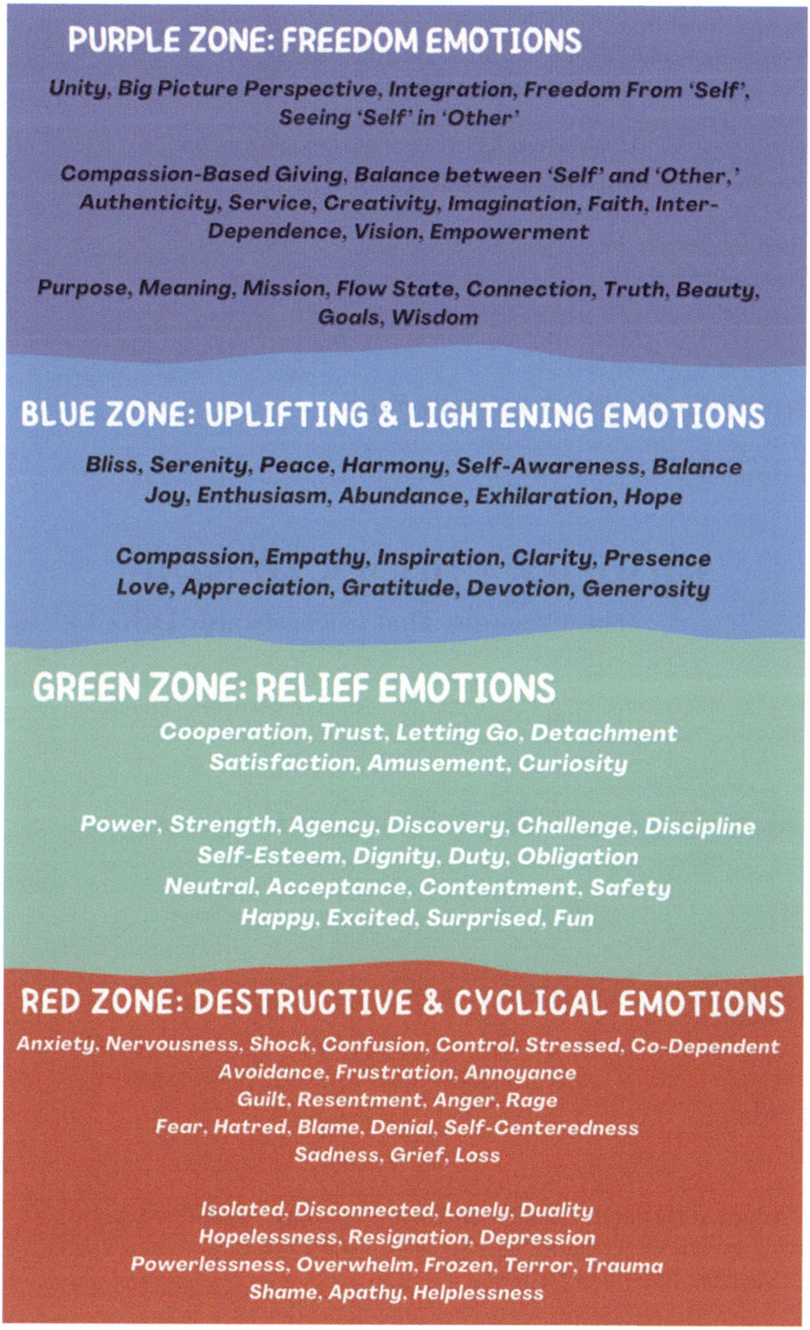

B. Adapted Rational Emotive Behavior Therapy (REBT) Exercises:
-Adapted and Simplified by Creator of HBMP, Sara Spowart, LMFT
Reframing Negative Beliefs Example:

Negative Identified Belief: *There's no reason to be happy.*
What is the benefit of this negative identified belief?
I Get More Attention from My Family and Others When I Feel Sad
What is the harm of this negative identified belief?
Feeling Bad, not Helping Mood or Wanting to Stay Sober
3 Positive Alternatives to Identified Belief:

(a) There is at least one reason to be happy
(b) Eventually there could be a reason to be happy
(c) I am mostly just hurting myself with this belief

C. Identity Circle: Which is Really *You*?

-Made by HBMP Creator, Sara Spowart, LMFT

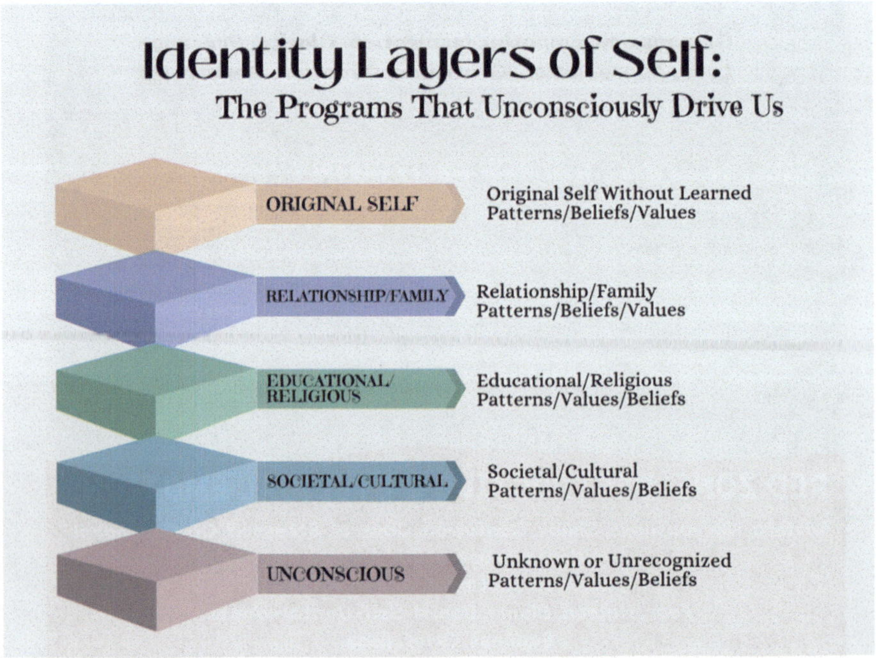

D. Adapted Rational Emotive Behavior Therapy (REBT) Exercise
-Made by HBMP Creator, Sara Spowart, LMFT
(1) Negative Identified Belief:

What is the benefit of this negative identified belief?

What is the harm of this negative identified belief?
3 Positive Alternatives to Identified Belief:

(a).
(b).
(c).

E. Compassion-Based Resiliency Chart

-Made by HBMP Creator, Sara Spowart, PhD, LMFT

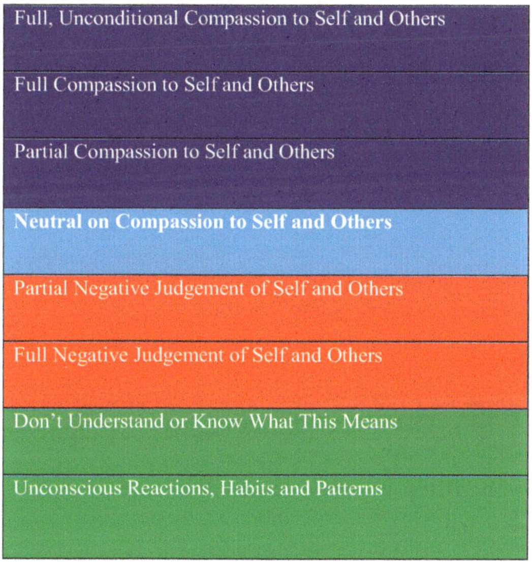

F. The Nervous System, Safety & Rest Exercise

Close Your Eyes and Sit in a Comfortable Position, and Maybe with Your Feet on the Floor

- *Take a deep breath in through your nose and out through your mouth*
- *Take another deep breath in through your nose and out through your mouth*
- *Take one more deep breath in through your nose and out through your mouth*
- *And as i count down from 5 to 1, feeling more and more relaxed, calm and at peace*
- *5–4 Feeling more relaxed*
- *4–3*
- *3–2 Calmer and calmer*
- *2–1 Feeling calm, relaxed and at peace*
- *Imagine that you are sitting near a grassy green field and peaceful forest*
- *Breath in peace and calm*
- *Breath out the feeling of support and safety*

- *Notice the breath in and out and the flow of the air*
- *Now, Imagine You Are Standing up and then Are Walking Towards the Forest*
- *As You Walk Towards the Forest, You Feel More and More Supported, Calm and at Peace*
- *Deep Breath in and Out, Allowing Yourself in This Moment to Be Safe and Supported*
- *Breathing in Support and Compassion*
- *Breathing Out Support and Compassion*
- Then imagine that you are wearing a back-pack full of rocks, and these rocks are everything and anything that is weighing you down, causing you trauma, stress, pain and fear
- You walk over to a lake in the forest, and this lake dissolves any and all the rocks in your backpack
- One by one throwing these rocks into the lake, and they melt and dissolve away
- 3
- 2
- And 1
- These rocks melt and dissolve away completely
- And throwing your backpack into the lake now, and it dissolves away completely
- And you feel lighter and lighter, more and more at peace and at ease
- Deep breath in and out,
- Imagining yourself sitting in this forest by the lake
- And you are filled with rest
- Your head, neck and shoulders…in this moment, it is safe to rest
- Your arms and hands ….in this moment, it is safe to rest
- Your torso, heart, chest, and stomach…rest
- Your back, hips, legs and feet…all rest
- And you breath in a feeling of rest and relaxation, and breath out
- Knowing that in this moment, it is safe to rest, relax and experience some peace
- …

For Instructors of the Brief Trauma-Focused HBMP:

(1) Participate in all 3 sessions with a certified brief trauma-focused HBMP instructor and review the program, core concepts, course set-up, and activities.
(2) Please complete the Brief Trauma-Focused HBMP and all 3 sessions. Completing the program will help you to be ready to teach so you are familiar with and have a deep understanding of the material.
(3) Please read and reference all materials in the program and become familiar with the activities and the ongoing practice of them. This includes a comfortable use and regular application of all activities provided.

References

Alesane, A. (2022). Microfinance, livelihoods and poverty reduction in Ghana. Taylor & Francis.

Asnaani, A., Charlery White, S. A. R., Majeed, I., & Phillip, T. M. (2020). Trauma education and stigma reduction in global settings: An evaluation of the impact of a one-day trauma psychoeducation workshop with community stakeholders in the Caribbean Nation of Saint Lucia. *International journal of environmental research and public health, 17*(7), 2255.

Bika, Z., Subalova, M., & Locke, C. (2022). Microfinance and small business development in a transitional economy: Insights from borrowers' relations with microfinance organisations in Kazakhstan. *The Journal of Development Studies, 58*(1), 183–203. https://doi.org/10.1080/00220388.2021.1956472

Chikwira, C., Vengesai, E., & Mandude, P. (2022). The impact of microfinance institutions on poverty alleviation. *Journal of Risk and Financial Management, 15*(9), 393.

Clark, A. E., Flèche, S., Layard, R., Powdthavee, N., & Ward, G. (2017). The key determinants of happiness and misery.

Helliwell, J. F., Layard, R., & Sachs, J. D. (2017). *World Happiness Report 2017*. Sustainable Development Solutions Network. https://worldhappiness.report/ed/2017/

Helliwell, J. F., Layard, R., & Sachs, J. (Eds.). (2013). *World Happiness Report 2013*. UN Sustainable Development Solutions Network.

Helliwell, J., Layard, R., & Sachs, J. (2018). *World Happiness Report 2018*. Sustainable Development Solutions Network.

Helliwell, J. F., Layard, R., Sachs, J., & De Neve, J.-E. (Eds.). (2020). *World Happiness Report 2020*. Sustainable Development Solutions Network.

Hershler. (2021). *Looking at trauma: a tool kit for clinicians* (Hershler, Ed.). The Pennsylvania State University Press. https://doi.org/10.1515/9780271092287

Hock, R. S., Or, F., Kolappa, K., Burkey, M. D., Surkan, P. J., & Eaton, W. W. (2012). A new resolution for global mental health. *The Lancet, 379*(9824), 1367–1368.

Jones, R. B., Thapar, A., Rice, F., Beeching, H., Cichosz, R., Mars, B., & Simpson, S. A. (2018a). A web-based psychoeducational intervention for adolescent depression: Design and development of MoodHwb. *JMIR Mental Health, 5*(1), e8894.

Jones, R. B., Thapar, A., Stone, Z., Thapar, A., Jones, I., Smith, D., & Simpson, S. (2018b). Psychoeducational interventions in adolescent depression: A systematic review. *Patient Education and Counseling, 101*(5), 804–816.

Kabat-Zinn, J. (2021). The liberative potential of mindfulness. *Mindfulness, 12*(6), 1555–1563.

Kim-Prieto, C., Diener, E., Tamir, M., Scollon, C. N., & Diener, M. (2005). Integrating the diverse definitions of happiness: A time-sequential framework of subjective well-being. *Journal of Happiness Studies, 6*, 261–300.

Klussman, K., Curtin, N., Langer, J., & Nichols, A. L. (2022). The importance of awareness, acceptance, and alignment with the self: A framework for understanding self-connection. *Europe's Journal of Psychology, 18*(1), 120.

Korkmaz, Z. (2021). The effect of the schema therapy-based psycho-education program on the depression and happiness levels of teachers. *Humanistic Perspective, 3*(3), 720–736.

Lorenzetti, L. M., Leatherman, S., & Flax, V. L. (2017). Evaluating the effect of integrated microfinance and health interventions: An updated review of the evidence. *Health Policy and Planning, 32*(5), 732–756.

Marquez, J., & Main, G. (2021). Can schools and education policy make children happier? A comparative study in 33 countries. *Child Indicators Research, 14*, 283–339.

Martinez, J. (2015). Revisiting the Happiness Formula. *ETC A Review of General Semantics, 208–218*, 1.

McRae, K., & Gross, J. J. (2020). Emotion regulation. *Emotion, 20*(1), 1.

Mehrabi, Y., Ghazavi, Z., & Shahgholian, N. (2017). Effect of fordyce's happiness program on stress, anxiety, and depression among the patients undergoing hemodialysis. *Iranian Journal of Nursing and Midwifery Research, 22*(3), 190.

Mills, C. (2018). From 'invisible problem' to global priority: The inclusion of mental health in the sustainable development goals. *Development and Change, 49*(3), 843–866.

Mueser, Rosenberg, S. D., & Rosenberg, H. J. (2009). *Treatment of posttraumatic stress disorder in special population: a cognitive restructuring program* (First edition.). American Psychological Association.

Ortet, G., Pinazo, D., Walker, D., Gallego, S., Mezquita, L., & Ibáñez, M. I. (2020). Personality and nonjudging make you happier: Contribution of the Five-Factor Model, mindfulness facets and a mindfulness intervention to subjective well-being. *PLoS ONE, 15*(2), e0228655.

Ruducha, J., & Jadhav, M. (2018). A review of organizational arrangements in microfinance and health programs. *Journal of Global Health Reports, 2.*

Sachs, J. D., Layard, R., & Helliwell, J. F. (2018). *World happiness report 2018* (No. id: 12761).

Sachs, J. D. (2017). Restoring American happiness. *World Happiness Report, 2017*, 178.

Sachs, J. D. (2018). America's health crisis and the Easterlin paradox. *World Happiness Report, 218*, 146–159.

Sachs, J. D. (2019). Addiction and unhappiness in America. *World Happiness Report, 2019*, 122–131.

Santomauro, D. F., Herrera, A. M. M., Shadid, J., Zheng, P., Ashbaugh, C., Pigott, D. M., & Ferrari, A. J. (2021). Global prevalence and burden of depressive and anxiety disorders in 204 countries and territories in 2020 due to the COVID-19 pandemic. *The Lancet, 398*(10312), 1700–1712.

Séverin. (2021). Mali. *African Disability Rights Yearbook*, 7 https://doi.org/10.29053/24137138/2019/v7a8

Spowart, S. (2022). A path to happiness. In *Happiness and Wellness-Biopsychosocial and Anthropological Perspectives*. IntechOpen.

Spowart, S. (2024). Global happiness and humanitarian assistance. Springer Nature.

Srivastava, P., & Panday, R. (2016). Psychoeducation an effective tool as treatment modality in mental health. *The International Journal of Indian Psychology, 4*(1), 123–130.

Vahratian, A., Blumberg, S. J., Terlizzi, E. P., & Schiller, J. S. (2021). Symptoms of anxiety or depressive disorder and use of mental health care among adults during the COVID-19 pandemic—United States, August 2020–February 2021. *Morbidity and Mortality Weekly Report, 70*(13), 490.

Van Rooyen, C., Stewart, R., & De Wet, T. (2012). The impact of microfinance in sub-Saharan Africa: A systematic review of the evidence. *World Development, 40*(11), 2249–2262.

Whitworth, J. D. (2016). The role of psychoeducation in trauma recovery: Recommendations for content and delivery. *Journal of Evidence-Based Social Work, 13*(5), 442–451. https://doi.org/10.1080/23761407.2016.1166852

Wollburg, C., Steinert, J. I., Reeves, A., & Nye, E. (2023). Do cash transfers alleviate common mental disorders in low-and middle-income countries? A systematic review and meta- analysis. *PLoS ONE, 18*(2), e0281283.

World Health Organization. (2017). Depression and other common mental health disorders: global health estimates, *Google Scholar*.

World Health Organization. (2018). mhGAP operations manual.

World Health Organization. (2018). *Delivering global health security through sustainable financing: 26–27 July 2017, Seoul, Republic of Korea* (No. WHO/WHE/CPI/2018.38). World Health Organization.

World Health Organization. (2021). Suicide worldwide in 2019: global health estimates.

World Health Organization. (2022). World mental health report: transforming mental health for all. In *World mental health report: transforming mental health for all.*

Part II

Large-Scale Humanitarian Issues and Solutions

Food Insecurity in Humanitarian Assistance

4

Taylor Stone

Abstract

Nutrition is one of the foundations of health. Food insecurity leads to malnutrition, which impacts not only physical health but mental health as well. This is especially evident in populations facing humanitarian crises. There were over 35 million refugees in the year 2022 and this number continues to rise with natural disasters, global inflation, and various conflicts worldwide. Food insecurity exists universally, affecting low- and high-income countries. Refugees encounter additional complexities in nutrition not only due to humanitarian crises but also because of various systemic factors in their new countries. The purpose of this chapter is to provide insight on the many obstacles that refugees face regarding food security, and to promote possible solutions to improve health outcomes for these populations globally.

Keywords

Food insecurity • Displaced person • Humanitarian aid • Chronic disease • Public health

1 Introduction

A refugee is a person who has left their home to seek asylum in another country due to circumstances in their own country such as political unrest, violence, war, and other threats and they have a right to protection by another country (United Nations High Commissioner for Refugees, n.d.) They may be previously persecuted based on race, religion, political affiliation, culture, or other reasons. Over

T. Stone (✉)
University of South Florida in Tampa, Tampa, FL, USA
e-mail: taylor390@usf.edu

S. Spowart (ed.), *Global Happiness and Humanitarian Assistance*, Integrated Science 29, https://doi.org/10.1007/978-3-031-71789-5_4

half of the refugees originate from Syria (6.5 million), Ukraine (5.7 million), and Afghanistan (5.7 million) (United Nations High Commissioner for Refugees, n.d.). This paper will primarily focus on challenges and solutions for refugees in humanitarian aid, but it is important to note the differences between refugees, internally displaces persons, and asylum seekers. There were 35.3 million refugees in the year 2022, as well as 62.5 million internally displaced people, who seek refuge in other places, but do not necessarily cross international borders (United Nations High Commissioner for Refugees, n.d.). There are also 5.4 million asylum-seekers, who seek safety in another country, but are waiting for legal protection to become a refugee (United Nations High Commissioner for Refugees, n.d.). These are growing populations due to the many natural disasters and conflicts, so it is imperative for humanitarian aid workers and organizations to assess the health concerns of these large groups and not only assist in emergent situations, but to provide long-term solutions as well. Refugee populations have many challenges in their home countries, while traveling, and in their new host countries, so it is essential to outline these concerns and prevent them for future generations. While the first priority is to ensure the safety and security for such populations, there are many challenges refugees face, even after relocating to a new country. Over 76% of refugees are hosted in low- or middle-income countries, which may exacerbate the poor conditions of those being rehoused (United Nations High Commissioner for Refugees, n.d.). One major concern in populations receiving humanitarian aid is the lack of proper nutrition, which may lead to further health concerns in the future.

1.1 Nutrition Basics

Nutrition is essential for the health of all people globally. Not only does it promote the growth and development of children, but it improves immune systems, provides energy, and encourages overall quality of life (World Health Organization, n.d.). Healthy diets include those with plenty of vegetables, fruits, whole grains and protein, while being low in salt and fat (World Health Organization, n.d.). Also, diets rich in vitamins and minerals can control weight, blood sugar, blood pressure, and mental health (World Health Organization, n.d.). A person who consumes adequate carbohydrates, protein, and vitamins may experience enhanced cognitive function, resulting in improved mental health outcomes (Suarez-Lopez et al., 2023). Unfortunately, millions of people worldwide face food insecurity, which is not just a lack of food, but a decrease in nutritious options due to factors such as poverty, discrimination, or food swamps and food deserts (Feeding America, n.d.). Food insecurity can range from mild (decrease in access) to severe (starvation) (Oldroyd et al., 2022).

Many of the leading causes of death are diet-related non-communicable diseases (NCDs) including heart disease, cancers, and diabetes mellitus (World Health Organization (2020). Heart disease accounted for more than 10 million deaths, cancer caused over 900,000 deaths, and diabetes mellitus led to 300,000 fatalities, a 70% increase since 2000 (Elshahat & Moffat, 2020; Global Burden of Disease,

2019). Poor nutrition led to approximately 11 million deaths worldwide during the year 2017 (Global Burden of Disease, 2019). Of these deaths, 3 million were due to high intake of sodium, another 3 million were linked to insufficient consumption of whole grains, and 2 million were associated with a low intake of fruits (Elshahat & Moffat, 2020). Proper nutrition is important in preventing morbidity and mortality worldwide. This proves the significance of promoting healthy diets among refugees and other vulnerable populations in humanitarian aid settings. Global food insecurity is widespread, and refugees face additional factors contributing to malnutrition and related issues.

1.2 Food Insecurity

There are multiple obstacles refugees must face in their home country and while traveling. They may experience challenges such as separation from family, trafficking, lack of food, water, and shelter, trauma, poverty, and absence of proper medical care (National Child Traumatic Stress Network, n.d.). When refugees relocate, there may be difficulties with housing, transportation, culture, language and communication, access to resources, education, and healthcare (National Child Traumatic Stress Network, n.d.). Among the most significant problems refugees encounter during their journeys and upon arrival in a new country is the prevalence of food insecurity.

Most refugees resettle in countries with low or medium incomes where malnutrition rates are even higher due to economic challenges; however, refugees in high-income countries encounter similar challenges related to unfamiliar food systems and lack of nutritional variety to meet their specific needs (Khuri et al., 2022). In the United States alone, more than 34 million people, including 9 million children, are food insecure. (Feeding America, n.d.). It is not the effects of one individual, but of the entire system. Due to low household incomes and global inflation, many households in the United States had to choose between food and other necessities such as medical care, housing, utilities, and education (Feeding America, n.d.). Australia's food insecure population reached 22% or 4.6 million people, while Japan's food insecurity reached 16% or 19.8 million, Canada's population was 8% (1.9 million people), and Europe reached 9% (43.6 million people) (Pollard & Booth, 2019). These numbers increased after the COVID-19 pandemic and recent conflicts worldwide. Though food banks are predominantly utilized by those with severe food insecurity, attendance rates in these countries have risen up to 33% in some regions (Oldroyd et al., 2022). Though food banks are a great resource for emergent or short-term needs, there are still limitations to solving food insecurity. For example, food parcels may be low in meat, dairy, and micronutrients and they do not always provide culturally appropriate foods for all populations (Oldroyd et al., 2022). Therefore, refugee populations may be sustained temporarily by these food choices, but if this occurs long-term, there may be further consequences for them in the future.

Food security is not just about ending hunger, but about providing healthy, nutritious options to all populations. For refugees, food insecurity may be increased due to poor transportation, difficulty navigating the new environment, and cultural differences with foods (Steeves et al., 2022). These factors, as well as lack of proper healthcare in their new countries, may lead to chronic illnesses for adults and children alike. Refugees come from many different nations globally and may relocate to developing or developed nations including those in the Americas, Europe, and the Middle East. Depending on cultural differences between refugees and their host nations, there are various concerns with nutritional deficiencies.

2 Poverty

According to the UNHCR Global Trends data, 76% of refugees are relocated to low- and middle-income countries (United Nations High Commissioner for Refugees, n.d.). Refugees relocating from Africa have rates of food insecurity up to 85% (Steeves et al., 2022). Not only do low- and medium-income countries have greater rates of food insecurity, but they also have higher rates of fast-food consumption (Smith et al., 2022). This makes it more difficult for refugees who enter the country, as they may mirror the host nation's food habits. Though refugees relocate to new nations after challenges such as violence or disasters, they will not be without trials in their new countries. For example, many Afghan refugees in Pakistan met numerous obstacles with malnutrition and food insecurity. Pakistan is a low-income country with high poverty rates and overcrowding, leading to food insecurity for Afghan refugees (Fatima et al., 2023). Out of 150 Afghan women observed, 74% of which were underweight, and many had anemia as well as depression, fatigue, and diarrhea (Fatima et al., 2023). This can affect not only female refugees negatively but can cause concerns for their children as well. Reasons for Afghan malnutrition in Pakistan included impoverished conditions, low socioeconomic status, low education level, and cultural differences in diets (ie eating bread with every meal and drinking tea instead of water) (Fatima et al., 2023).

Though developed nations have a higher per capita income and Gross Domestic Product (GDP), there are still issues of food insecurity, especially in refugee and displaced populations. Many of these concerns are due to economic challenges, but they also face obstacles related to unfamiliar food systems and lack of nutritional variety to meet their specific needs (Khuri et al., 2022). These concerns often arise from poor transportation, difficulty navigating the new environment, and cultural differences with foods (Steeves et al., 2022). This proves difficult for host nations to provide proper tools for these populations. Many countries, such as the United States, Canada, and those in Europe have food banks to assist those with food insecurity, but this is a short-term fix (Oldroyd et al., 2022). These food banks may assist with hunger and emergent situations, but there also should be programs in place that address prevention of food insecurity, such as employment and education, specifically for vulnerable populations.

2.1 Geographic Differences

Refugees residing in the United States have difficulties with food security stemming from issues such as navigating unfamiliar surroundings, cultural disparities (for example, the inability to find halal foods), transportation limitations, lack of access to healthy food in grocery stores, and limited availability of food bank resources (Goliaei et al., 2023). Many refugees have to use public transportation, such as the bus, due to limitations in income or in obtaining state driver's licenses. There may not be buses or street cars available in their areas, so walking may be the only method of transportation, limiting the options of grocery stores. It may be difficult to navigate in the new country, and grocery stores may be unfamiliar, with confusing packaging and food labels. This makes it problematic to adhere to proper food choices and can lead to increased food insecurity. Many refugees prefer smaller, international grocery stores to enhance their familiarity, and they tend to spend more money on rice and meat than fruits and dairy products (Burge & Dharod, 2018). They also may find vegetables to be expensive, so many families grow their own in their backyards; however, this method tends to fall short of providing sufficient nutrients (Burge & Dharod, 2018). The overwhelming experience of a different grocery store, area, or new labels can lead refugees to make poor diet choices, leading to improper nutrition. It is important not only to educate refugees on geography, grocery stores, and food labels, but for local grocery stores to provide culturally appropriate food choices for all religions and backgrounds. It is also essential to oversee the prices of healthy food in stores located within areas of these vulnerable populations to ensure they may acquire such items within their budget constraints. This may be a more difficult process in low-income countries, but it is essential for the health of these populations.

Refugees may have a difficult time navigating a new healthcare system as well. If they do not have the proper resources to seek care, they are at risk for chronic illnesses. Refugees may avoid seeking care for conditions such as obesity or diabetes due to factors such as language barriers, unfamiliarity with the healthcare system, discomfort with various healthcare providers, or conflicts between work schedules and appointment times (Ofosu et al., 2022). For example, when refugees enter Germany, they cannot seek care for the first year unless it is under the category of acute illness or pain (Biddle et al., 2019). This system discourages refugees from healthcare for chronic conditions, leading to further issues in the future. Refugees in Germany self-reported poorly controlled chronic illnesses including mental illness and emphasized the lack of access to primary care and specialists in the country. If these issues are uncontrolled in refugee populations, this leads to further overuse of the German health system in the future.

Refugees require education on the importance of healthcare, especially for those with chronic disorders, but adaptations should be made for these vulnerable populations as well. For example, they should be provided with translators and doctors who are aware of their cultural practices. This not only will enable the refugees to be properly educated in their health but will provide comfort and encouragement for their next visit. It is essential to reveal barriers to healthcare and mitigate those to ensure proper health promotion for refugees.

2.2 Diet

A well-balanced diet serves as the cornerstone for both physical and mental health. Dietary patterns differ globally, and maintaining a nutritious diet can pose challenges following relocation. For example, Burmese refugees who relocated to the United States were knowledgeable on the importance of a healthy diet, but various fruits and vegetables were not easily accessible for them (Myo et al., 2023). Educating refugee populations on balanced diets may not be necessary for ensuring food security; however, ensuring access to appropriate and nutritious food options is crucial for their well-being. Only 45% of the Burmese refugees ate the proper number of fruits and vegetables and 86% of them reported lack of access to healthy foods at preferred stores (Myo et al., 2023). The ease of access to healthy options such as fruits and vegetables has a large impact on populations, regardless of previous diets and knowledge of nutrition. Money is also a factor for eating healthy. Foods such as rice and pasta tend to be cheaper, but they do not provide proper protein or micronutrients compared to foods such as meats and vegetables (Amstutz et al., 2020).

Many diets are reflective of religion or cultural practices. Acculturation is when a refugee faces challenges, especially dietary practices, in their new country, such as cultural or navigational differences, leading to a change in their habits, lasting generations (Elshahat & Moffat, 2020). Many refugees in the United States increased their fast-food consumption and decreased their consumption of vegetables, lean meats, and whole grains (Elshahat & Moffat, 2020). Typically, those with higher rates of acculturation in the United States made unhealthy food choices upon arrival. The biggest barriers were lack of nutritional knowledge, decreased resources for infant nutrition, and poor tasting fruits and vegetables in the United States (Elshahat & Moffat, 2020).

Not only do refugees have a difficult time-consuming healthy food, but they may find it easier and cheaper to eat unhealthy food. There are many factors that influence food patterns, but people who relocate to Western countries such as Canada and the United States increase their intake of processed foods, sugar, fat, and salt, leading to heart disease and diabetes (Li et al., 2023). Food swamps are areas with an abundance of fast-food choices and unhealthy food options, and they are common in the United States, especially in areas of low socioeconomic status. These restaurants typically have large portions of easily accessible, unhealthy food that may be provided quickly. Despite being high in calories, sugars, and fats, individuals may perceive these foods as more convenient and cost-effective compared to the effort and expenses associated with grocery shopping and food preparation. Therefore, populations in low-income areas are more susceptible to poor nutrition and food insecurity. The influence of food marketing starts at an early age, so nutritional education should be initiated early in life.

Children may have life-long disorders from malnutrition, so it is key to teach them how to make nutritious choices as soon as possible, ideally in early elementary ages. Children who receive healthy snacks and proper dietary education have higher rates of nutrients such as Vitamin K, zinc, calcium, and magnesium, as well as fiber, protein, and saturated fat (Diab El Harake et al., 2018). By introducing such methods at a young age, refugees may learn how to eat healthy options, even in their new countries. This is especially important in children as it will impact their health throughout their lifetime.

Adolescents are especially prone to weight gain and obesity due to dietary changes in their new countries. Many refugee adolescents entered the United States and while physical activity decreased, they had increased consumption rates of sugary drinks, milk, and meat (Sastre & Haldeman, 2020). Refugees who entered the United States had higher rates of obesity than the United States' average, which can lead to health problems such as diabetes and heart disease (Sastre & Haldeman, 2020). It is important for refugee adolescents to be taught moderation for foods such as sugary drinks and snacks. Dietary interventions may be taught in school to promote healthy diet and exercise.

2.3 Disabilities

Another population to highlight is people with disabilities. Over 1 billion people have disabilities worldwide and vulnerable populations such as this have a more difficult time with transportation, education, and healthcare, leading to an increased rate of food insecurity or malnutrition (Hernandez-Vasquez et al., 2023). People with disabilities may face discrimination and may be unable to work, leading to greater rates of poverty. Most of these disabled populations are in low- or middle-income countries and the populations with the greatest representation of food insecurity were elderly, females, chronic illnesses, or those unemployed (Hernandez-Vasquez et al., 2023). NGOs and public health officials should collaborate with refugees to determine skills and level of education to promote autonomy and employment. This will also provide them with a sense of accomplishment, leading to greater mental health outcomes. It is important to be inclusive of refugees, especially when introducing them to the host country's communities, and disabled persons deserve the same level of respect. Many refugees, especially those who are disabled, had food insecurity issues prior to relocation, so the new country should find ways to assess and treat malnutrition.

3 Consequences

There are many nutritional deficiencies in refugees, which increases the chance of chronic disease development in children and adults. Much of the food assistance provided, especially in the Middle East, lacks nutritious options, primarily consisting of grains and flour (Basu et al., 2018). Over 40% of the refugees in the Middle East receive food aid, so millions of people are not receiving proper nourishment due to budget constraints (Basu et al., 2018). As a result, diabetes and heart disease are the leading chronic conditions and causes of death for Palestinian refugees (Basu et al., 2018). Nutrition not only impacts physical health, but mental health as well.

3.1 Physical Health

Adults who are food insecure are more likely to face obesity, insulin resistance, and high cholesterol (Smith et al., 2022). These conditions can lead to chronic diseases such as anemia and diabetes, exacerbated by the replacement of nutritious food with less expensive, unhealthy foods full of salt and saturated fats (Feeding America, n.d.). Many refugees had increased consumption of salt, leading to high blood pressure and an increased consumption of fatty foods, leading to high cholesterol (Khuri et al., 2022). Refugees also may have an imbalance in nutrients such as vitamin A, leading to vision problems, zinc, leading to an impaired immune system, iodine, leading to thyroid disorders, and vitamin C, leading to delayed wound healing or even scurvy (Centers for Disease Control & Prevention, 2019). If food aid decreased grains by 8.5% and increased fruits and vegetables to match, there would be a reduction in Body Mass Index (BMI), blood pressure, sodium and fat consumption, and cholesterol, leading to a decrease in diabetes, high blood pressure, heart disease, and end-stage renal disease (ESRD) (Basu et al., 2018). This shows the significance diet has on nutritional status as well as chronic diseases.

Proper nutrition is important for growth and may set a child up for a more successful, healthy future. In children, food insecurity can lead to health issues such as developmental delays, and asthma (Feeding America, n.d.). Refugee children were more likely to have stunted growth and many refugees lacked micronutrients such as calcium, iron, and vitamin D, leading to anemia (Khuri et al., 2022). Prolonged anemia in children and adolescents may lead to reproductive concerns and fatigue later on in life (Centers for Disease Control & Prevention, 2019). It is important to address these issues at a young age so children can grow into healthy adults. It is also vital to teach children how to make nutritious choices at a young age to improve their health long-term. Poor nutrition and chronic diseases may also impact the mental health of children and adults.

3.2 Mental Health

Refugee mental health is impacted by many factors including history of conflict or natural disasters, separation from their homes, and even food insecurity. Refugees have higher rates of mental health disorders in both high- and low-income countries (Kamelkova et al., 2023). This is exacerbated by impoverished conditions, inability to find work, and food insecurity. Malnutrition can result in mental health concerns such as anxiety, depression, insomnia, and focus (Kamelkova et al.,

2023). These issues may lead to further difficulties with work and other tasks, leading to a downward spiral of mental and physical concerns. Also, those who are food insecure face many social issues including feelings of humiliation, vulnerability, and dependency on the government (Pollard & Booth, 2019). They may consume a greater number of salts and fats as a coping mechanism to such stress, leading to poor nutrition as well (Smith et al., 2022).

Malnutrition can lead to mental health concerns such as anxiety and even aggression in children (Feeding America, n.d.). Poor food choices and consumption of fast-food can increase violent behaviors in children, and research has shown an increase in mental health disorders such as depression because of this (Smith et al., 2022). Poor nutrition and chronic diseases may also impact the mental health of children and adults. Typically, food aid in humanitarian settings is meant for temporary circumstances but can sometimes lead to long-term dependency. By providing healthier options in refugee camps and at food banks, rates of chronic diseases may be decreased once refugees are officially rehoused.

4 Potential Solutions

This chapter outlined the significance of nutritional deficiencies on chronic disorders in refugees. Whether refugees are in low- or high-income countries, they are at a higher risk of nutritional deficiencies. This is exacerbated in refugee populations with disabilities. Not only do refugees have pre-existing nutritional deficiencies from their travels or from camps, but they also have difficulties upon resettlement as well. Food insecurity in refugees after resettlement may be due to lack of healthy, culturally appropriate options, confusion with navigating the new area, increased fast-food restaurants, or lack of resources such as employment or education. Refugees have an increase in salt and fat and a decrease in vegetable intake upon arrival to the United States. This leads to higher rates of obesity, as well as chronic diseases such as high blood pressure, heart disease, diabetes, and mental illnesses. It is important to note that many refugees endure hardships including violent events, trafficking, and other traumatic experiences, so they may underreport or downplay food insecurity and its resulting conditions (Goliaei et al., 2023). If countries do not have appropriate access to healthcare for refugees, these chronic conditions continue. Therefore, it is important to further research this topic, especially using longitudinal studies.

Many studies found nutritional deficiencies in refugees, but more research is required to compare refugees before and after entering their new country, as well as chronic conditions later in life. If possible, performing basic measurements of height and weight as well as diet and lifestyle assessments would be beneficial before leaving the home country and upon entering the new country. Completing this task may pose a challenge as refugees typically seek refuge in other countries due to violence, leaving little time to establish these baseline measurements. However, if time-permitting, in-depth assessments would be valuable to determine the impact of travel on nutritional status. This is important research as it will provide information before and after relocation, as well as identify gaps in refugee health statuses.

A needs assessment would first be conducted for the refugee population in the new country. This would outline the priorities for the population. Upon entering their new countries, refugees should undergo an immediate medical evaluation conducted by physicians and nutritionists. These exams would include both mental and physical health categories. A past medical history should be performed including history of infections, hospitalizations, immunizations, and surgeries, as well as any new medical concerns while traveling (Centers for Disease Control & Prevention, 2019). A thorough medical examination may be required as malnutrition can show in hair, dentation, and other systems, but a simple measurement of malnutrition, especially in children, is height and weight (Centers for Disease Control & Prevention, 2019).The nutritional assessment may also include previous food logs, dietary restrictions, supplements, and for infants, formulas or breastfeeding schedules (Centers for Disease Control & Prevention, 2019). Labs should be performed during this initial assessment, if possible, followed by additional tests as needed, taking into consideration age and any abnormal laboratory studies. Labs that may be performed, based on host nation's capabilities, would include albumin and a complete blood count to determine anemia status, as well as vitamins such as folate and vitamin D (Centers for Disease Control & Prevention, 2019). Assessment of fat and muscle mass can also be a strong indicator for nutritional status, and this is performed through tricep thickness test, skin fold test, hand-grip strength, or DEXA scans (Bharadwaj et al., 2016). Though these tests are accurate and beneficial in identifying cases of malnutrition, they may be unnecessary and no single factor in such assessments is conclusive. Therefore, it is important to look at individual cases, when possible, and provide solutions tailored to each refugee.

Upon relocation to refugee camps or their new homes, food parcels may be provided for emergency consumption to prevent further malnutrition. Unfortunately, this method may not be used as a long-term solution because many food parcels provided do not always have culturally appropriate foods or foods high in micronutrients, meats, or dairy products (Oldroyd et al., 2022). Humanitarian aid organizations should collaborate with fresh-food distributors to enhance these options for temporary purposes. Other populations may require education on topics such as nutrition, diet related NCDs, local grocery store practices, food labels, cooking, and breastfeeding. These may be taught in classroom settings with hands-on courses in cooking healthy foods with proper seasonings. These classes would enhance their familiarity with the local area, empowering them to prepare nutritious meals in their new country while maintaining their culture. The classes and community meals also promote socialization and allow refugees to maintain their cultural norms (Amstutz et al., 2020). Breastfeeding programs can also be advantageous in ensuring proper nutrition for infants while providing supplemental formula as needed. This would enhance growth and development at a young age, preventing diet related NCDs in the future. Gardening is another skill that could be helpful in providing autonomy for refugees, as well as providing healthy foods for their diets. These community-based programs would be beneficial and can be started in refugee camps or in their communities.

Needs assessments are required for these populations and detailed planning and evaluation will be essential in the successful implementation of such humanitarian aid programs. Depending on the program, humanitarian aid organizations have to collaborate with various partners to assist these populations. Stakeholders may include Registered Dietitians (RDs), Certified Lactation Consultants (CLDs), agricultural specialists, medical providers, public health officials, and other educational experts. Logistical planning is also required to ensure the correct supplies are delivered by local volunteer organizations, NGOs, and governmental programs. Lastly, evaluation is a key step in this process. Regular monitoring should be done with refugee feedback to identify areas of improvement. It is also important to note that refugees are more likely to thrive in educational nutrition programs when they have strong support systems and access to culturally appropriate food while barriers to learning include language differences, unfamiliar environments, and lack of class attendance (Gough et al., 2020).

There are many solutions to the problems outlined in this chapter, but they require extensive research, medical assessments, planning, and collaboration with stakeholders. Given the uniqueness of each refugee population and host country, it is crucial to assess the needs of the population and determine priorities to combat food insecurity and malnutrition. Some populations primarily require education on nutrition, whereas others need assistance with navigating grocery stores and transportation. It is up to the host country, healthcare officials, public health officials, and NGOs to perform assessments on the refugees and tailor solutions to specific populations for chronic disease prevention. These programs should be flexible and look at all factors including socioeconomic status, level of education, cultural norms, and physical activity. With such programs in host countries, refugees can lead longer, healthier lives.

5 Ethical Considerations

Refugees have the same rights as any other population, so ethical considerations are of the utmost importance in these cases. First, refugees must have access to basic needs such as food, water, shelter, and proper sanitation. This also includes the right to safety and dignity. This can be difficult to maintain, especially in emergency settings, due to the influx of refugees and rationing of resources, but these basic needs must be a minimum of care for large populations. Second, there should be no discrimination based on race, gender, age, religion, ethnicity, class, or nationality. Marginalized groups must also receive equal access to resources and care. Humanitarian organizations must have respect for the local area and practices but know when to bring extra help or resources. Involving the local population and the refugees may provide autonomy and empowerment, allowing them to provide insight into decisions. Cultural norms must be considered, especially regarding research practices, healthcare, and nutrition. This also includes proper communication and education provided to refugees.

6 Conclusion

This chapter identified common themes amongst refugee groups with nutrition and chronic diseases. Refugees are prone to food insecurity and malnutrition for various reasons including unfamiliarity with the geographic location or with grocery stores, language and communication barriers, food labels, dietary practices including an uptake in meat and sugary drinks and snacks, lack of culturally appropriate foods, and disabilities. These nutritional deficiencies are observed via physical assessments (dentation, hair, height, and weight), labs (hemoglobin, iron, vitamin D, and albumin), and through other tests. Refugees of all ages and backgrounds have increased rates of nutritional deficiencies for various reasons including traumas, dietary practices, or lack of food options. It is important for public health officials to collaborate with NGOs in ensuring proper assessments not only upon arrival to new countries, but prior to leaving their home countries, if possible. This will provide crucial information for further research studies. By continuing research on refugee populations, public health officials may uncover gaps in existing literature and current public health processes. While many public health policies and programs are in place regarding refugee nutrition, there is a need for ongoing research to shape the future of humanitarian aid.

References

Amstutz, D., Goncalves, D., Hudelson, P., Stringhini, S., Durieux-Paillard, S., & Roulette, S. (2020). Nutritional status and obstacles to healthy eating among refugees in Geneva. *Journal of Immigrant and Minority Health, 22*(6), 1126–1134. https://doi.org/10.1007/s10903-020-01085-4

Basu, S., Yudkin, J. S., Berkoqitz, S. A., Jawad, M., & Millett, C. (2018). Reducing chronic disease through changes in food aid: A microsimulation of nutrition and cardiometabolic disease among Palestinian refugees in the Middle East. *PLOS Medicine*. https://doi.org/10.1371/journal.pmed.1002700

Bharadwaj, S., Ginoya, S., Tandon, P., Gohel, T. D., Guirguis, J., Vallabh, H., Jevenn, A., & Hanouneh, I. (2016). Malnutrition: Laboratory markers vs nutritional assessment. *Gastroenterol Rep, 4*(4), 272–280. https://doi.org/10.1093/gastro/gow013

Biddle, L., Menold, N., Bentner, M., Nost, S., Jahn, R., Ziegler, S., & Bozorgmehr, K. (2019). Health monitoring among asylum seekers and refugees: A statewide, cross-sectional, population-based study in Germany. *Emerging Themes in Epidemiology*. https://doi.org/10.1186/s12982-019-0085-2

Burge, C., & Dharod, J. M. (2018). What are the nutrition education needs of refugees: Assessment of food choices, shopping, and spending practices of South-Asian refugees in the USA. *Journal of International Migration and Integration, 19*, 555–564. https://doi.org/10.1007/s12134-018-0565-1

Centers for Disease Control and Prevention. (2019, October 23). *Nutrition and growth*. https://www.cdc.gov/immigrantrefugeehealth/guidelines/domestic/nutrition-growth.html

Diab El Harake, M., Kharroubi, S., Hamadeh, S. K., & Jomaa, L. (2018). Impact of a pilot school-based nutrition intervention on dietary knowledge, attitudes, behavior, and nutritional status of Syrian refugee children in the Bekaa Lebanon. *Nutrients, 10*(7), 913. https://doi.org/10.3390/nu10070913

Elshahat, S., & Moffat, T. (2020). Dietary practices among Arabic-speaking immigrants and refugees in Western societies: A scoping review. *Appetite.* https://doi.org/10.1016/j.appet.2020.104753

Fatima, M., Nosheen, F., Afzaal, M., Islam, F., Noreen, R., Imran, A., & Ali, Y. A. (2023). Nutritional and health status of Afghan refugee women living in Pubjab: A cross-sectional study. *Food Science Nutrition, 11*(6), 2872–2882. https://doi.org/10.1002/fsn3.3267

Feeding America. (n.d.). Hunger and food insecurity. https://www.feedingamerica.org/hunger-in-america/food-insecurity#:~:text=A%20definition%20of%20food%20insecurity,people%20can%27t%20afford%20food

Feeding America. (n.d.). *Compromises and coping strategies.* https://www.feedingamerica.org/hunger-in-america/impact-of-hunger

Global Burden of Disease. (2019). Health effects of dietary risks in 195 countries, 1990–2017: A systematic analysis for the Global Burden of Disease study 2017. *Lancet, 393*, 1958–1972. https://doi.org/10.1016/S0140-6736(19)30041-8

Goliaei, Z., Gonzalez, M., Diaz Rios, K., Pokhrel, M., & Burke, N. J. (2023). Post-resettlement food insecurity: Afghan refugees and challenges of the new environment. *International Journal of Environmental Research and Public Health, 20*(10), 5846. https://doi.org/10.3390/ijerph20105846

Gough, J., Wengreen, H., Nur, H., & Archuleta, M. (2020). P55 providing nutrition education to refugees: Successful strategies and barriers to success in current programs. *Journal of Nutrition Education and Behavior, 52*(7), 41–42. https://doi.org/10.1016/j.jneb.2020.04.101

Hernandez-Vasquez, A., Reategui, A. B., Sanchez-Davila, K., & Vargas-Fernandez, R. (2023). Association between disability and unmet food needs in the Venezuelan migrant and refugee population: Analysis of a population-based survey, 2022. *Nutrients, 15*(7), 1663. https://doi.org/10.3390/nu15071663

Kamelkova, D., Strømme, E. M., & Diaz, E. (2023). Food insecurity and its association with mental health among Syrian refugees resettled in Norway: A cross-sectional study. *Journal of Migration and Health.* https://doi.org/10.1016/j.jmh.2023.100173

Khuri, J., Wang, Y., Holden, K., Fly, A. D., Mbogori, T., Mueller, S., Kandiah, J., & Zhang, M. (2022). Dietary intake and nutritional status among refugees in host countries: A systematic review. *Advances in Nutrition, 13*(5), 1846–1865. https://doi.org/10.1093/advances/nmac051

Li, C., Carolino, E., & Sousa, J. (2023). Dietary acculturation and food habit changes among Chinese immigrants in Portugal. *Nutrients, 15*(8), 1886. https://doi.org/10.3390/nu15081886

Myo, H. W., Hosler, A. S., Schell, L. M., Allsopp, M. A., & Reid, K. (2023). Factors associated with fruit and vegetable consumption among Burmese refugees. *Public Health Nutrition, 26*(6), 1264–1270. https://doi.org/10.1017/S13680023000125

National Child Traumatic Stress Network. (n.d.). *About refugees.* https://www.nctsn.org/what-is-child-trauma/trauma-types/refugee-trauma/about-refugees

Ofosu, N. N., Luig, T., Chiu, Y., Mumtaz, N., Yeung, R. O., Lee, K. S., Wang, N., Omar, N., Yip, L., Aleba, S., Maragang, K., Ali, M., Dormitorio, I., & Campbell-Scherer, D. (2022). Understanding the bigger picture: Syndemic interactions of the immigrant and refugee context with the lived experience of diabetes and obesity. *BMC Public Health, 22*, 345. https://doi.org/10.1186/s12889-021-12305-3

Oldroyd, L., Eskandari, F., Pratt, C., & Lake, A. A. (2022). The nutritional quality of food parcels provided by food banks and the effectiveness of food banks at reducing food insecurity in developed countries: A mixed-method systematic review. *Journal of Human Nutrition and Diabetics, 35*(6), 1202–1229. https://doi.org/10.1111/jhn.12994

Pollard, C. M., & Booth, S. (2019). Food insecurity and hunger in rich countries—It is time for action against inequality. *International Journal of Environmental Research and Public Health, 16*(10), 1804. https://doi.org/10.3390/ijerph16101804

Sastre, L. R., & Haldeman, L. (2020). Diet, physical activity and weight-related behaviors, changes, and risks with newly-arrived (<1 year) immigrant and refugee adolescents (ages 12–17). *Journal of Immigrant and Minority Health, 22*, 282–290. https://doi.org/10.1007/s10903-020-00970-2

Smith, L., Barnett, Y., Lopez-Sanchez, G., Skin, J., Jacob, L., Butler, L., Cao, C., Yang, L., Schuch, F., Tully, M., & Koyangagi, A. (2022). Food insecurity (hunger) and fast-food consumption among 180 164 adolescents aged 12–15 years from sixty-eight countries. *British Journal of Nutrition, 127*(3), 470–477. https://doi.org/10.1017/S0007114521001173

Steeves, B. A., Hollis-Hansen, K., McElrone, M., Nur, H., & Landry, M. J. (2022). Supporting food and nutrition security among migrant, immigrant, and refugee populations. *Journal of Nutrition Education and Behavior, 55*(2), 83–84. https://doi.org/10.1016/j.jneb.2022.12.003

Suarez-Lopez, L. M., Bru-Lana, L., & Marti-Vilar, M. (2023). Influence of nutrition on mental health: Scoping review. *Healthcare, 11*(15), 2183. https://doi.org/10.3390/healthcare11152183

United Nations High Commissioner for Refugees. (n.d.). *Figures at a glance.* https://www.unhcr.org/us/about-unhcr/who-we-are/figures-glance#:~:text=How%20many%20refugees%20are%20there,under%20the%20age%20of%2018

United Nations High Commissioner for Refugees. (n.d.). *What is a refugee?* https://www.unrefugees.org/refugee-facts/what-is-a-refugee/

World Health Organization (2020, December 9). *The top 10 causes of death.* https://www.who.int/news-room/fact-sheets/detail/the-top-10-causes-of-death

World Health Organization. (n.d.). *Nutrition.* https://www.who.int/health-topics/nutrition#tab=tab_1

School-Based Mental Health Interventions: Global Case Studies and Solutions

5

Bailey Rae Brannan

Abstract

Children and teenagers are particularly vulnerable to the current global mental health crisis. Large-scale, school-based interventions are potentially effective for addressing this global challenge. A majority of countries worldwide require compulsory schooling and therefore provide the greatest potential to assist large numbers of minors in mental illness prevention. Mental illness often includes co-morbidities such as substance abuse, and physical and sexual abuse. Therefore, school-based mental health interventions have the potential to prevent future addiction and abuse that children may later experience as adults. Different intervention approaches as well as barriers and challenges are explored.

Keywords

Mental health • School-Based interventions • Global health • Child mental health • Prevention

1 Introduction

The global mental health crisis is affecting people of all ages. However, children and teenagers are uniquely vulnerable in that adverse mental health events could result in negative life courses. Intervention strategies designed to prevent the onset of mental health conditions and to treat conditions that already persist show promise in curbing negative life outcomes in adulthood. Schools provide ideal settings for offering these interventions to the most people possible. Schools can

B. R. Brannan (✉)
University of South Florida, Tampa, FL, USA
e-mail: brannan.baileyrae@gmail.com; bbrannan@usf.edu

S. Spowart (ed.), *Global Happiness and Humanitarian Assistance*, Integrated Science 29, https://doi.org/10.1007/978-3-031-71789-5_5

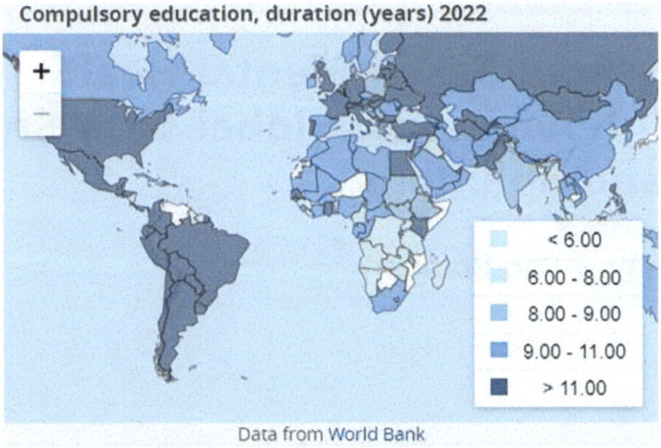

Fig. 1 Shaded map of countries that possess education requirement, courtesy of the World Bank (World Bank Open Data, 2023)

successfully link all involved parties— students, families, community members, interventionists, and mental health professionals.

2 Increasing Influence

Around the world, the majority of individuals between the ages of five and eighteen have some exposure to the public school system. According to the 2022 data provided by The World Bank (World Bank Open Data, 2023), the majority of countries engage in compulsory education for at least some period of time during childhood and adolescent development. Given the legal requirement to attend school in many countries, school-based interventions offer the greatest promise for reaching a high number of students (Fig. 1).

Additionally, interventionists strive to reach students during their critical developmental window. Researchers found that earlier intervention shows greater promise in preventing abuse or other adverse events (Thompson et al., 2022). In Erika Thompson's particular study, her team focused on mental health interventions on school-aged children between the approximate ages of eight and ten (i.e., third through fifth grade in the U.S. school system). Though older students may demonstrate more content knowledge overall, the younger students showed higher levels of growth. Thus, earlier intervention is essential to protecting the highest number of individuals. Further research supports early interventions predicting higher levels of mental and emotional stability as well (Adams et al., 2018).

3 Global Evidence for Supporting Youth in the School System

While local schools provide one of the best venues for mental health interventions, the proposed methods of intervention differ. Some methods are prevention-focused, in that the goal is to avoid the onset of mental health conditions. Other methods

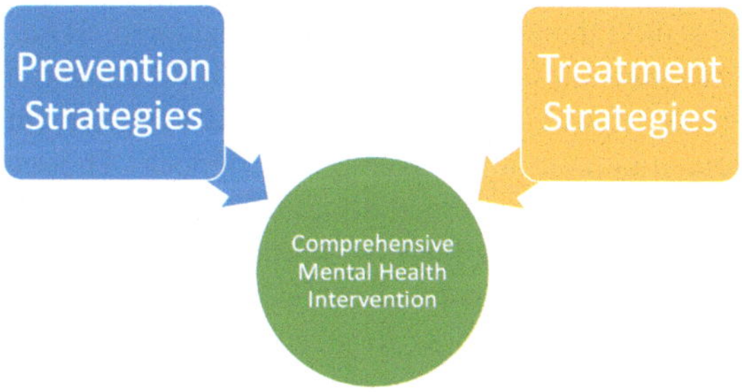

Fig. 2 Coupling of prevention and treatment strategies provides a well-rounded school-based intervention program

are treatment-focused, in that the goal is to manage mental health conditions that already persist in the student body. Both types of approaches have their advantages, as outlined below. However, a truly comprehensive school-based intervention system will lean into both pillars of strategy (Fig. 2).

3.1 Prevention Strategies

Often, mental health challenges occur with comorbidities, or the coupling or tripling of mental health conditions. Some common comorbidities include substance abuse disorder, depression, post-traumatic stress disorder (PTSD) and anxiety (Jystad et al., 2021). In preventing substance abuse or events that could inspire the onset of other comorbidities, the effects of the main mental health challenge are mitigated. Instances of abuse—both psychical and sexual—are also tied to the later onset of mental health challenges including PTSD, anxiety, and depression (Adams et al., 2018). The outcomes of abuse on mental health are unpredictable, both in severity and the time at which the condition presents itself. Therefore, it is beneficial for school employees to promote comprehensive preventative education to proactively prevent possible sources of trauma.

3.1.1 Physical and Sexual Abuse Prevention

In the United States, researchers found success in an intervention designed to educate third through fifth grade students on the signs of sexual abuse (Thompson et al., 2022). These researchers specifically studied the *Play It Safe!* curriculum in upper elementary school classrooms, but the full curriculum offers scaffolded lessons from pre-kindergarten through twelfth grade. By high school, students typically can recognize advances from older or inappropriate individuals. However, they are less skilled at recognizing and preventing dating violence or other negative interactions with their peers. This scaffolded curriculum provides the opportunity for consistent preventative education and comprehensive tactics for recognizing, responding to, and reporting on instances of abuse (Thompson et al., 2022).

In Indonesia, researchers found success in preparing young children for recognizing and preventing sexual abuse (Wulandari et al., 2022). They tested their novel intervention, *Program Prevensi Pelechan Seksual Berbasis Sekolah (P3SBS)* and measured the effectiveness via the adapted *'What If' Situation Test* intervention on first-grade children. The program shows educational effectiveness, and researchers predict it will empower students to advocate for themselves in an effort to prevent traumatic and adverse experiences. Though first grade students are young, and some are concerned about discussing these sensitive topics with children, it is valuable to arm children with knowledge before abuse can occur. If educators wait until the age of typical sexual education curriculum (i.e., adolescence), they might miss a critical window for preventative measures.

Adverse childhood experiences, especially those related to abuse, predict rates of re-victimization in adulthood (Ports et al., 2016). The most impactful interventions must begin at younger ages. Early integration of abuse prevention programs offers the best chance of preventing abuse in children and re-victimization in adulthood. In preventing these traumatic and adverse experiences, interventionists can also prevent the onset of mental health conditions and comorbidities, including depression, anxiety, substance misuse/dependency, and PTSD.

3.1.2 Resisting Drugs

Substance abuse disorder arises as a common comorbidity with other mental health conditions. Recreational drug usage often exacerbates symptoms, complicates the effectiveness of prescribed medications, or disguises the mental health concern that necessitates treatment. In preventing drug misuse, the treatment of various mental health conditions is more streamlined and effective. Many school-based interventions address drug abuse. Physical education curriculum frequently embeds substance abuse education, and schools even implement established programs like *Drug Abuse Resistance Education (D.A.R.E.)* taught my law enforcement officers.

Additional drug resistance programs, like the *Ho'ouna Pono* that was implemented in an American school district, even provide opportunities for classroom teachers to deliver the curriculum (Okamoto et al., 2019). In this delivery model, teachers are eligible to provide the intervention after completing a one-day training course. Although this method places some increase in the teachers' workloads, they are supported by ongoing training and resources through a teacher login portal. Teachers are additionally compensated with continuing education credit for completing the training. These supports and incentives help motivate teachers to present important intervention programs that may otherwise be out of their comfort zones.

3.1.3 Cultivating a Sense of Belonging: Promoting Friendship and Inclusivity

Making friends serves as a positive predictor for school success and social adjustment and wellbeing (Danby et al., 2012). Researchers in Australia found that students require opportunities to request participation in activities, collaborate meaningfully, and reach out to others and invite them to participate in activities as necessary. Susan Danby and her team acknowledge the vital role teachers, coaches, and club leaders can play in facilitating these opportunities.

Promoting a sense of belongingness in schools allows for the creation of friendships and higher levels of wellbeing. Feelings of belongingness can stem from positive behavioral interventions and supports (PBIS) (Smith Ramey et al., 2023), affiliation with a team or subgroup beyond grade level (e.g., the "red team" of seventh graders), or comfortable collaborative opportunities. Danby's team also found that adjustment to school could be facilitated through a schoolmate that is already an established friend or relative, somewhat like a mentor. This opens up the possibility for a mentoring program, where new, vulnerable, or potentially all students could be partnered with a mentor. The mentor would provide the first interpersonal connection and allow for an easier transition to new friendships.

Friendships are crucial in promoting emotional growth and stability. In Vietnam, researchers apply this knowledge through the *Happy House* intervention (Tran et al., 2023). Interventionists attempt to cultivate students' feelings of belongingness, but the intervention requires modifications to reach statistically significant results. However, the intervention produced high levels of students' self-efficacy, which is associated with more positive feelings towards school in general.

To combat feelings of loneliness, researchers in the United States recruited high school participants (i.e., students between the ages of 14 and 19) to participate in online lessons in the *Heartfulness Institute's Self-Care program* (Iyer et al., 2023). They found significant decreases in students' loneliness scores over the 28-day intervention. This intervention is delivered online, so it is feasible to implement in schools without requiring additional mental health personnel. Correcting feelings of loneliness will allow students to feel more accepted in their school environment and promote better emotional health.

3.1.4 Positive Psychology as Prevention

In the Netherlands, researchers show promise in assisting students and their psychological wellbeing via positive psychology school-based interventions (Kennes et al., 2023). The intervention of focus is mindfulness training—*Think Happy-Be Happy*. In this intervention, students participate in eight 45-min training sessions. The session length approximates the length of a class period, which assists in its implementation in a school system. Researchers found significant improvement in emotional and psychological well-being following the intervention. However, six-months post-intervention, the results did not maintain significant lasting effects. Thus, the results emphasize a need for continued mindfulness intervention to sustain student wellbeing and prevent the onset of mental health challenges. A one-off intervention is not enough to curb the rise of mental health conditions. Consistency is key in developing positive mental framework, resilience, and enduring coping mechanisms (Kennes et al., 2023; Tran et al., 2023).

3.2 Treatment Strategies

By providing treatment in the school system, treatment becomes more accessible to those that are marginalized (Renshaw & Phan, 2023). Many students face barriers to mental health treatment, such as physical accessibility, affordability, and lack of multi-tiered support—requiring cooperation from both families and the school system to expand support. Integrating treatment with schools will increase access to students with a demonstrated need for assistance.

3.2.1 Mandatory In-school Screenings

United Kingdom-based researchers studied the perceived attitudes towards in-school mental health screening (Williamson et al., 2022). They found that generally, parents would accept the implementation of screenings, so long as they are completed in a sensitive manner and there is follow-through on the next steps. Sometimes, parents of children in need of these screenings have barriers to access and feel frustrated with the lack of assistance (Williamson et al., 2022). Thus, while identification of a mental health issue is the first step towards treatment, schools must then connect identified students and their families with additional, accessible resources.

3.2.2 Partnerships with External Resources

Partnerships with external resources provide a crucial link between students in need of additional assistance and the accessibility of aid. Increasing the number of mental health professionals in the school building places a major strain on resources. However, partnering with community providers increases access with fewer personnel. With a partnership in place, it is crucial that communication with the students' families is prioritized (Smith Ramey et al., 2023). This helps facilitate trust between the involved parties, especially since the nature of mental health issues remains delicate. In situations where students require the next tier of mental health services (e.g., individual counseling or prescribed medications), the school can serve as the liaison between parties. Parents can receive assistance in navigating the mental healthcare system, while students receive interventions that allow for successful completion of school.

3.2.3 Positive Psychology and Coping

Positive psychology may serve as a treatment method as well. Anne Kennes and her research team (2023) demonstrated decreases in Dutch adolescents' inattention, hyperactivity, and relational conflicts post-intervention (Kennes et al., 2023). In the *Think Happy-Be Happy* mindfulness intervention, students learned strategies for resilience and coping. These strategies are especially useful in managing interpersonal conflict or internal turmoil—both of which could easily transform into larger issues without self-employed de-escalation approaches. In Vietnam, the *Happy House* intervention educates students on effective coping strategies (Tran et al., 2023). Post-intervention, researchers found a significant decrease in the levels of clinically depressive symptoms amongst students. *Happy House,* through six weekly 90-min lessons, teaches students how to manage stress and negative feelings. These treatment-focused interventions help students manage their symptoms.

3.3 A Note on Special Populations

Certain sub-groups of the general school-aged population require special levels of care in executing mental health interventions. Curricula may need additional levels of scaffolding to achieve broader levels of comprehension. Some populations may require supplemental modules or lessons to cover special topics pertaining to sexuality and/or those with physical or mental disabilities. For students in the sexual and gender minority, interventions are particularly useful in teaching them effective coping mechanisms. Researchers in Nigeria studied the coping mechanisms that these individuals employ when experiencing challenges related to their mental health, including thoughts of suicide (Rodriguez-Hart et al., 2023). Some coping mechanisms are healthy, but others, like avoidance, are not healthy. When applying interventions in the school setting, interventionists should take care to focus on empowerment and confidence. Additional coping strategies may need to be addressed with these populations.

Researchers in the United Kingdom (Kelly et al., 2023) addressed the unique concerns about students with special needs. Though many existing prevention and treatment programs have the surface-level appearance of being inclusive, the programs tend to lack effective accommodations and adaptations to ensure full engagement from these students. The UK-based team specifically adapted the *Speak Out Stay Safe* curriculum and modified comprehension assessments after the program delivery. They found that, with proper accommodations—including modified pre-/post-tests, additional teacher assistance in the classroom, previewing the material before program presentation, and video/role-play follow-up educational methods—students with special needs can engage in preventative programs effectively. Students with special needs pose unique vulnerabilities, and it is especially imperative that these students are educated on how to advocate for themselves.

4 Barriers and Challenges

Historically, relationships between the school system and families have not always been smooth or trusting (Williamson et al., 2022). Schools regularly engage in outreach initiatives to improve relationships, but the initiatives do not always have the greatest impact. Perhaps, providing mental health screening and intervention services at the school could provide a method to strengthen the relationship between the school system and the families it serves (Williamson et al., 2022). Attendance also poses an issue. Even in schools dedicated to implementing mental health interventions, student attendance is largely out of their control. Yet, absences may decrease the effectiveness of the intervention and/or decrease student motivation in acquiring resilience and coping skill education (Kennes et al., 2023).

The rigorous pacing of the core curriculum serves as an additional barrier to implementing mental health initiatives during the school day. In many school systems, students diligently prepare for end-of-year testing to determine academic progress and future course placement. In some countries, these tests have higher stakes than others. Thus, the situation creates a cascading effect, in that students faced with the most academic pressure have the least amount of time to participate in mental health interventions, despite mental health interventions playing a key role in developing qualities such as resilience, coping, and tenacity—which are quintessential traits for surviving rigorous curricula. Budgeting school minutes for these interventions may pose a difficult task for school administrators. However, the reward of clearer-minded and well-adjusted students who develop lifelong skills and assistance through mental health interventions far surpasses the cost of some educational minutes. Perhaps, if school officials are concerned with the potential gouge to curriculum time, they may seek support from local policymakers and legislators to increase the school day by the appropriate amount of time.

An additional challenge is the personnel shortage. In some cases, school systems are constrained by strict budgets that do not allow for additional student support employees. In other cases, rural and less desirable school districts struggle to attract qualified candidates. In either case, people often look to teachers to fill these positions and set aside a day of their normal classroom routines to address mindfulness or abuse-prevention topics. While this seems to address the personnel shortage at the surface level, this model is severely problematic (Thompson et al., 2022). To start, many teachers do not feel comfortable addressing sensitive topics or qualified enough to deliver a specialized lesson (e.g., mindfulness) outside of their specialty area (Lu et al., 2022; Thompson et al., 2022).

Thus, external delivery via trained professionals is often required. However, even with visiting interventionists tackling the bulk of prevention-centered education or treatment techniques, teachers and those with daily student contact must receive some basic training in order to accurately recognize signs of mental health challenges and to appropriately contact further help and resources for the student (e.g., the social worker, the school out-patient referral program, etc.). Though prior research suggests that early intervention is critical—especially in prevention methods (Thompson et al., 2022)—some raise concerns about the age appropriateness of the lessons (Lu et al., 2022). What are age-driven boundaries for prevention education? Often, if someone is old enough to recognize abuse for what it is, it is too late to educate them from a prevention standpoint. Treatment options are certainly appropriate when scaffolded for all ages. However, prevention interventions, which often focus on sensitive abuse-prevention topics, remain a concern.

5 Overcoming Barriers: from Theory to Practice

In practice, the school system is the most effective way to access young people between the ages of five and eighteen. This access occurs without prejudice, stigma, or hindrance due to life's circumstances. All students are eligible for the primary tier of classroom intervention. Through these interventions, teachers and others involved with children can identify those requiring extra tiers of mental health support. Access to these additional tiers hinges on the school system's ability to connect with external community resources. It is essential that the tier-one intervention material is regularly embedded and scaffolded for appropriateness based on age and potential vulnerabilities during that developmental period for students. Research suggests that the earlier abuse occurs, the more severe the symptoms of mental health issues (Adams et al., 2018). Mental health issues are most likely to arise if abuse occurs during childhood, primarily between the ages of six and twelve. However, the severity and duration of the abuse also play a role in the onset of mental health issues.

Thus, in the prevention-oriented intervention method, early implementation of effective programs is crucial in generating the highest levels of success in protecting youth. Consistency is also key to successful school-based interventions. Even with statistically effective strategies, results do not persist six months after implementation (Kennes et al., 2023). Instead of isolated assemblies or limited-time interventions, tier one mental health interventions should be regularly integrated into the weekly, if not daily, curriculum. Interventions may have a place in physical education classes, homeroom periods, or a new class dedicated to mental and emotional wellbeing.

Ultimately, schools hold a considerable deal of power and influence in terms of disseminating information on proactivity, protection, prevention, coping, and treatment for a variety of mental health issues. Aside from direct in-school interventions, schools also have the ability to engage with and educate community members on the same issues and pathways for help. Additionally, schools provide a key link between students, their families, and outside resources, perhaps through partnerships with local clinics and mental health practices. Schools are accessible to nearly all community members and stakeholders involved in child wellbeing. Utility and accessibility make the local school an ideal meeting place for community education and involvementin (Fig. 3).

Fig. 3 Branches of school system's influence for intervention

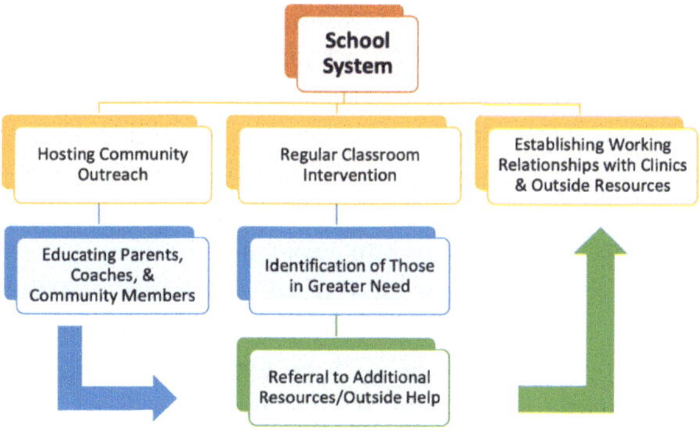

6 Accessibility and Adaptability

When implementing school-based interventions on a global scale, stakeholders must ensure the cultural relevance of their programs of choice. While it is advantageous to learn from successes in other countries, the models may need adjustment to fit the unique needs of a different country's population. For example, in Brazil, educational institutions took part in the popular D.A.R.E. program to reduce substance abuse. While the program is popular and generally effective in the United States, researchers in Brazil are noting the opposite effect in that the desire for substance abuse is increasing (Valente & Sanchez, 2022). This illustrates the importance of adapting established international programs to the specific needs of the young people in the country of interest. Interventionists in Indonesia found success in adapting abuse prevention curriculum to their language and culture (Wulandari et al., 2022). The established *'What If' Situation Test* was modified to the correct language and for cultural relevance so it could be used as an assessment method. Additionally, the Vietnamese *Happy House Adolescent Program* intervention was culturally and linguistically adapted from the initial Australian intervention, *Resourceful Adolescent Program* (Tran et al., 2023). These adaptations increase the effectiveness of the programs.

Interventions must also be adapted appropriately to the age group. For example, in the Netherlands, researchers referenced an established mindfulness intervention for adults and transformed it into a similar strategy for adolescents (Kennes et al., 2023). Some of the modifications included shortened practice exercises, given concerns for participation, focus, and stamina. These modifications were designed to increase effectiveness for the target age group, but they also make the method more appropriate and usable in the classroom setting. Furthermore, curricula concerning mental health interventions must be appropriately adapted to fit the needs of those in special populations (Kelly et al., 2023). Even with cultural modifications, prevention and treatment strategies are not a one-size-fits-all. For true success, interventionists must consider the unique needs of sub-populations.

In terms of accessibility, sometimes students choose to seek support from peers instead of trusted adults. Comprehensive intervention programs include suggestions for speaking out on a friend's behalf, beyond tools for empowering oneself. Programs that encourage friends to look out for one another help minimize the gap between those who are impacted by mental health issues and those who are seeking help (Kelly et al., 2023). Text-message reporting methods have shown some promise in increasing participation in students seeking help (Ortiz & Smith, 2023). The text-message program was initially designed for students to report instances of bullying or people at risk of self-harm, but the same method can likely be applied to students seeking other forms of help. Increasing accessibility to students through methods such as texting and online applications may increase the number of students who receive help.

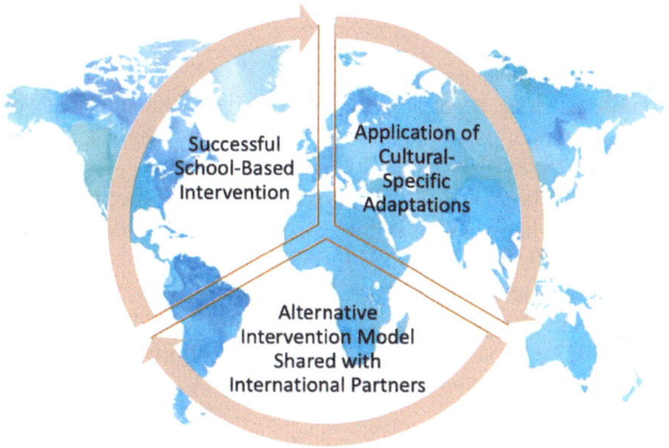

Fig. 4 Global facilitation of school-based mental health interventions and adaptations

7 Conclusions: Moving Forward

Although multiple successful mental health interventions—both prevention-oriented and treatment-oriented—exist, it remains crucial that whatever intervention in place receives careful and regular review. In order to stay relevant and effective, school officials, policymakers, and interventionists hold a duty to evaluate the effectiveness and rigor of their programs (Thompson et al., 2022). The nature of intervention will certainly change over time, and monitoring the strategies for intervention and altering them as necessary will help provide the greatest amount of assistance to those in need.

Schools certainly provide the greatest opportunity to reach a substantial number of the world's youth and teenagers. However, interventions within the four walls of the school are not enough. Those involved in mental health interventions implore school systems to expand their outreach (Lu et al., 2022), perhaps by hosting educational seminars for the public or partnering with extracurricular activity coaches. When schools serve as the community liaison between students and families in need and mental health officials, barriers to treatment are lowered, and students can receive the mental health help they seek.

Ultimately, we can all learn from one another (Lu et al., 2022). Many dedicated professionals are working diligently to address the global mental health crisis and its effects on young people. As we learn from others and modify the effective strategies with our cultural and language requirements, we can create and share new versions of successful interventions. By combining prevention-focused and treatment-focused interventions—minding the special needs of sub-groups in the population—stakeholders can make a change in the state of the global mental health crisis (Fig. 4).

References

Adams, J., Mrug, S., & Knight, D. C. (2018). Characteristics of child physical and sexual abuse as predictors of psychopathology. *Child Abuse Neglect, 86*, 167–177. https://doi.org/10.1016/j.chiabu.2018.09.019

Danby, S., Thompson, C., Theobald, M., & Thorpe, K. (2012). Children's strategies for making friends when starting school. *Australasian Journal of Early Childhood, 37*(2), 63–71. https://doi.org/10.1177/183693911203700210

Iyer, R. B., Vadlapudi, S., Iyer, L., Kumar, V., Iyer, L., Sriram, P., Tandon, R., Morel, Y., Kunamneni, H., Narayanan, S., Ganti, A., Sriram, S., Tandon, R., Sreenivasan, S., Vijayan, S., & Iyer, P. (2023). Impact of the Heartfulness program on loneliness in high schoolers: Randomized survey study. *Applied Psychology Health and Well-Being, 15*(1), 66–79. https://doi.org/10.1111/aphw.12360

Jystad, I., Bjerkeset, O., Haugan, T., Sund, E. R., & Vaag, J. (2021). Sociodemographic correlates and mental health comorbidities in adolescents with social anxiety: The young-HUNT3 study, Norway. *Frontiers in Psychology, 12*, 663161–663161. https://doi.org/10.3389/fpsyg.2021.663161

Kelly, B., Farrelly, N., Batool, F., Kurdi, Z., & Stanley, N. (2023). Speak out, stay safe: Including children with special educational needs and disabilities in an evaluation of an abuse prevention programme. *Child Abuse Review Chichester England 1992*. https://doi.org/10.1002/car.2816

Kennes, A., Lataster, J., Janssens, M., Simons, M., Reijnders, J., Jacobs, N., & Peeters, S. (2023). Efficacy of a school-based mental health intervention based on mindfulness and character strengths use among adolescents: A pilot study of think happy-be happy intervention. *Journal of Happiness Studies, 24*(2), 677–697. https://doi.org/10.1007/s10902-022-00611-5

Lu, M., Barlow, J., Meinck, F., & Wu, Y. (2022). Prevention alone is not enough: Stakeholders' perspectives about school-based child sexual abuse (CSA) prevention programs and CSA research in China. *Journal of Interpersonal Violence*. https://doi.org/10.1177/0886260520959630

Okamoto, S. K., Kulis, S. S., Helm, S., Chin, S. K., Hata, J., Hata, E., & Lee, A. (2019). An efficacy trial of the Ho'ouna Pono drug prevention curriculum: an evaluation of a culturally grounded substance abuse prevention program in rural Hawai'i. *Asian American Journal of Psychology, 10*(3), 239–248. https://doi.org/10.1037/aap0000164

Ortiz, R. R., & Smith, A. (2023). Assessing the feasibility of a text message intervention to promote bystander intervention to adolescents. *Journal of School Violence, 22*(4), 1.

Ports, K. A., Ford, D. C., & Merrick, M. T. (2016). Adverse childhood experiences and sexual victimization in adulthood. *Child Abuse Neglect, 51*, 313–322. https://doi.org/10.1016/j.chiabu.2015.08.017

Renshaw, T. L., & Phan, M. L. (2023). Using implementation reporting to advance culturally sensitive and equity-focused mindfulness programs in schools. *Mindfulness, 14*(2), 307–313. https://doi.org/10.1007/s12671-023-02068-w

Rodriguez-Hart, C., Bradley, C., German, D., Baral, S., Ononaku, U., Dimlong, O. T., Crowell, T. A., Charurat, M., & Nowak, R. G. (2023). Building that strong energy: An exploration of stigma coping strategies among sexual and gender minorities in Nigeria. *Stigma and Health Washington D.c., 8*(2), 223–231. https://doi.org/10.1037/sah0000319

Smith Ramey, J., Lilley, S., Duis, M., & Volk, F. (2023). Depressed, disconnected, and distraught: School-based mental health intervention for rural youth. *Journal of Rural Mental Health, 47*(4), 240–247. https://doi.org/10.1037/rmh0000240

Thompson, E. L., Zhou, Z., Garg, A., Rohr, D., Ajoku, B., & Spence, E. E. (2022). Evaluation of a school-based child physical and sexual abuse prevention program. *Health Education Behavior, 49*(4), 584–592. https://doi.org/10.1177/1090198120988252

Tran, T. D., Nguyen, H., Shochet, I., Nguyen, N., La, N., Wurfl, A., Orr, J., Nguyen, H., Stocker, R., & Fisher, J. (2023). School-based universal mental health promotion intervention for adolescents in Vietnam: Two-arm, parallel, controlled trial. *Global Mental Health, 10*, e69–e69. https://doi.org/10.1017/gmh.2023.66

Valente, J. Y., & Sanchez, Z. M. (2022). Short-term secondary effects of a school-based drug prevention program: cluster-randomized controlled trial of the Brazilian version of DARE's Keepin' it real. *Prevention Science, 23*(1), 10–23. https://doi.org/10.1007/s11121-021-01277-w

Williamson, V., Larkin, M., Reardon, T., Ford, T., Spence, S. H., Morgan, F., & Creswell, C. (2022). Primary school-based screening for childhood mental health problems and intervention delivery: A qualitative study of parents in challenging circumstances. *Emotional and Behavioural Difficulties, 27*(4), 267–279. https://doi.org/10.1080/13632752.2022.2122285

World Bank Open Data. (2023). *Compulsory education, duration (years)*. https://data.worldbank.org/indicator/SE.COM.DURS?end=2022&most_recent_year_desc=false&start=2022&type=shaded&view=map

Wulandari, M. D., Hanurawan, F., Chusniyah, T., Hidayat, M. T., Rahmawati, F. P., Sayekti, I. C., & Bakhtiar, F. Y. (2022). Integration of a sexual abuse prevention programme in the first-grade Indonesian curriculum to improve children's self-protection. *Child Abuse Review Chichester England, 31*(2), 1. https://doi.org/10.1002/car.2723

Part III

Special Populations in Humanitarian Assistance

Gender Perspectives on Water, Sanitation, and Hygiene in Low- and Middle-Income Countries

6

Madison Weaver

Abstract

Inadequate access to safe, clean drinking water and appropriate sanitation and hygiene services and facilities (WASH) imposes a significant public health and human rights issue on many populations, especially in low- and middle-income countries. Poor access to WASH contributes to exposure and suffering from significant preventable disease and death, can hinder social and economic development, and impacts the overall well-being and quality of life of individuals and communities. While the impacts are widespread, women and girls face a disproportionate burden from WASH issues. This can be linked in parts to the reality of gender inequality for women and girls and in their specific biological needs. This assessment analyzes the various challenges and risks to the health, safety, and social and economic well-being of women and girls in relation to WASH. Eliminating detrimental WASH exposures and outcomes on women and girls will require utilizing an intersectional gender-transformative perspective. Gender-transformative approaches to WASH programming and policy presented in the current literature are explored here. These methods aim to transform the harmful gender dynamics that work to construct the discussed challenges and risks faced by women and girls. Through exploring gender-transformative approaches in WASH, it is proposed that harmful gender structures can be redressed to promote and protect the health, development, empowerment, and dignity of women and girls globally.

Keywords

Water, sanitation, and hygiene • Lower- and middle-income • Gender inequality • Women and girls • Gender-transformative approach

M. Weaver (✉)
College of Public Health, University of South Florida, Tampa, FL, USA
e-mail: mlweaver24@gmail.com

S. Spowart (ed.), *Global Happiness and Humanitarian Assistance*, Integrated Science 29, https://doi.org/10.1007/978-3-031-71789-5_6

1 Introduction

In 2022, an estimated 2.2 billion people lacked access to safe drinking water, 1.5 billion people were without basic sanitation services, and 2 billion people did not have access to handwashing facilities with soap (United Nations [UN], 2024). Lacking safe and accessible water, sanitation, and hygiene (WASH) imposes a significant burden on many communities, particularly in low- and middle-income countries (LMIC)—poor WASH conditions account for an estimated 1.4 million deaths each year, constrain the management and prevention of infectious diseases, especially diarrheal disease, exacerbate childhood malnutrition and stunting, hinder social and economic development, increase the risks for violence, create lost opportunities for education and work, and more (World Health Organization [WHO], 2019). WASH programming and policies are key public health targets for humanitarian aid and development in LMICs, with the goal of ensuring equitable access to water, sanitation, and hygiene—one of the most basic human needs and rights—for all (Centers for Disease Control and Prevention [CDC], 2022; Office for the Coordination of Humanitarian Affairs [OCHA], 2017).

2 Gender and WASH

Gender Definitions and Terms

What is Gender? According to the United Nations Development Programme (UNDP) (2010), gender can be described as the socially constructed opportunities, responsibilities, expectations, relationships, and powers associated with the different gender groups. As it is socially constructed, gender changes over time and varies from society to society. The defined attributes and positions of gender often invoke systematic inequality and discrimination

What are Gender-Transformative Approaches? Gender-transformative approaches aim to address the structural and social root causes of gender inequality. A gender-transformative approach is concerned with making changes in policy, services and systems, distribution of resources, behaviors, beliefs, norms, and more to remedy gender inequalities, remove structural barriers, and empower disadvantaged populations (Marcus et al., 2022)

Marginalized groups, especially women and girls, are disproportionately impacted by lacking access to safe and appropriate WASH. This is linked to systematic inequalities and discrimination from both the social constructs of gender and the biological needs of women and girls such as menstruation, pregnancy, lactation, and menopause. The opportunities, responsibilities, expectations, relationships, attitudes, needs, and powers of gender impede women's and girls' access to a most basic need and human right—WASH. Through exploring gender-transformative approaches in WASH programming and policy, as well as all areas of humanitarian action, it is proposed that harmful gender structures can be redressed to promote and protect the health, well-being, empowerment, and dignity of women and girls globally.

Note This assessment discusses only several challenges women and girls may experience in LMICs relating to WASH, these topics represent trends throughout the literature. It is important, however, to draw attention to the additional WASH experiences and needs among women and girls, briefly discussed or not discussed here including lactation, formula and complimentary feeding, caregiving and domestic work, menopause, menstruation, marital status, hand hygiene knowledge, disability status, age/life stage, and humanitarian emergencies.

2.1 Challenge: Water Collection

It is well documented that women and girls in many LMICs are disproportionately responsible for WASH, serving as the primary users, collectors, providers, and managers of the household or community water supply. Women and girls are estimated to be responsible for collecting water in 8 out of 10 households without water supplies on site (UN Women, 2018).

Collecting water presents numerous risks to the physical and psychosocial health, well-being, and livelihoods of women and girls. Women and girls who have to travel to gather water from distant locations spend an estimated average of one hour on water collection and maintenance activities every day (200 million collective hours every single day) (United Nations International Children's Emergency Fund [UNICEF], 2016a). Consequently, women lose time for caregiving, domestic tasks, contributing to agricultural production and food security, social interaction, education, and income/business endeavors, all of which can enhance autonomy, self-worth, dignity, and potential (UNICEF, 2016b; Swedish International Development Cooperation Agency [SIDA], 2019). Furthermore, during the journey to collect water, women and girls are at risk of physical injury, fatigue, violence, harassment, stress, and anxiety (WHO, 2023).

However, while women and girls typically hold the greatest responsibility and face significant related consequences, they are yet to have a representative role in WASH-related decision-making (UN Women, 2018).

2.1.1 School Attendance and Completion

In households or communities where there is no access to on-site water, children, especially girls, often help their mothers with water collection. This additional responsibility can lead to missed school days and incomplete education.

Girls are estimated to miss a total of 443 million school days each year due to water collection and water-related illnesses caused by inadequate WASH (UNDP, 2006). Moreover, the burden of water collection placed on girls contributes to the disproportionate completion of school between boys and girls. According to UNICEF (2015), 1 in 4 girls do not complete primary school, compared to only 1 in 7 boys who do not complete their education.

2.1.2 Safety and Violence

The burden of water collection not only disrupts women's and girls' activities and opportunities for personal improvement and prosperity but also increases their vulnerability to sexual and physical harassment and violence. This violence and harassment may be experienced when women and girls are travelling away from the community to collect water, putting themselves into possibly unsafe and unprotected environments. Tallman et al. (2022) have also documented the increased incidence of intimate partner violence experienced by women when they are unable to fulfill their domestic water collection duties.

The threat of violence during water collection puts many women and girls at risk of serious short and long-term physical and psychosocial consequences, including wounds, fractures or broken bones, infection, unwanted pregnancy, chronic pain, vaginal bleeding or pelvic pain, distress, anxiety, depression, post-traumatic stress disorder, shame, anger, and social disengagement (U.S. Department of Health and Human Services [HHS], 2021; Kimutai et al., 2023).

Unfortunately, there is significant under-documentation of both the quantitative and qualitative incidence of violence and harassment events among women and girls seeking to meet the water needs of their families and communities. Reliable data is widely unavailable. The gendered and sociocultural aspects of violence create complexities in data collection and the incorporation of reporting systems into WASH programming—due to the sensitive nature of this topic women and girls may feel shame, or fear consequences such as discrimination, stigmatization, and isolation when/if they would report such events (Sommer et al., 2014).

2.2 Challenge: Sanitation and Hygiene Resources

Proper sanitation and hygiene facilities promote health by allowing individuals to dispose of waste, use the latrine for urinating or defecating, and practice hygiene such as bathing, handwashing, and menstrual hygiene management (MHM) safely and appropriately (CDC, 2022).

The lack of water and sanitation in households and places such as schools, healthcare facilities, workplaces, and markets forces women to navigate challenging and even personally threatening public conditions to find a place to urinate, defecate, bathe, and manage menstruation.

2.2.1 Health and Hygiene Behaviors

As of 2020, it was estimated that only 44% of rural households have safely managed sanitation. Without access to household WASH facilities, as is typical in peri-urban and rural settlements of LMICs, individuals likely utilize shared community facilities that may not meet the basic needs of women and girls (Sultana & Crow, 2000; WaterAid, 2015).

Women and girls may feel unsafe or ashamed when using public, shared community sanitation and hygiene facilities. Latrines and bathing places are often located in public, visible spaces, and may lack safety measures such as doors, partitions/screens, locks, or proper lighting. Additionally, they may not provide appropriate resources for menstrual hygiene (Dickin & Gabrielsson, 2023). Socio-cultural and gender beliefs and norms may dictate the use of public latrines and hygiene facilities. While men typically face no social pressures when urinating, bathing, or defecating, many norms dictate that women's bodies should not be seen during these actions, and they even should not be seen entering latrine and hygiene facilities by men (MacArthur, 2023; Human Rights Watch, 2017; Jilali, 2021). As a result, women and girls may be forced to alter their sanitation and hygiene behaviors in ways that put their health and safety at risk:

- To avoid using public latrines or hygiene facilities during the day, many individuals wait to bathe and hold their urges to urinate or defecate until the nighttime when there is more privacy to use these facilities (Caruso et al., 2017; Jalali, 2021; Routray et al., 2015).
- Women and girls may travel outside of the community to fields, forests, bodies of water, or other open spaces to practice open urination or defecation if they cannot/do not want to utilize community facilities because of constraints (Caruso et al., 2017; Jalali, 2021).
- Women and girls may control their water and food consumption to reduce the need to urinate or defecate at specific times throughout the day or night (Jalali, 2021).
- Irregular bathing may be practiced by women and girls when they must exercise this personal hygiene practice in public bathing facilities (Jalali, 2021; Sahoo et al., 2015).

Although these behaviors may, in the short-term, make women and girls feel more at ease with the increase in privacy and perceived safety, they pose serious and threatening risks. These behavior changes practiced by women and girls to avoid latrines and hygiene facilities, practice open defecation and urination, and refrain from eating and drinking pose adverse health outcomes. These include outcomes such as chronic constipation, fecal impaction, distress and anxiety, feelings of shame and indignity, risk of infection, dehydration, and malnutrition (Hirve et al., 2015; WaterAid, 2015). Whether using public facilities or practicing behaviors to avoid them, women and girls may also face potentially unsafe environments where they may experience violence and harassment, posing short and long-term physical and psychosocial impacts. See Sect. 2.1.2.

2.2.2 School Sanitation and Hygiene Resources

Sanitation and hygiene infrastructure in schools can significantly impact children's health, well-being, and educational experiences. Clean, safe, and appropriate WASH facilities ensure that students can fully participate in school, especially adolescent girls who require resources for MHM. However, only an estimated 51% of schools have access to adequate and safe water resources on the premises and only 45% of schools have adequate and separate sanitation facilities for boys and girls (UNICEF, 2015; McMichael, 2019).

Lacking access to WASH in schools increases the vulnerability to educational interruptions, such as missed school days and noncompletion. When girls do not have access to resources including safe water for washing themselves or their menstrual clothes, gender-separate latrine facilities, safe menstrual products, and proper disposal systems, they are more likely to have lower attendance and higher dropout rates compared to boys (SIDA, 2019). According to UNICEF (2015), qualitative interviews and questionaries conducted among school-aged girls in LMICs found that more than 50% of the girls who dropped out of school reported that it was in direct relation to a lack of poor water, unclean sanitation facilities that did not provide privacy, and inability to access menstrual products and clothing changes.

As with behavioral changes reported in Sect. 2.2.1, when schools have no toilet facilities and girls are faced with the choice of using public community facilities or practicing open defecation, some girls may decide to hold their urges or limit food and drink consumption to delay the need to urinate or defecate. These behavior changes can result in adverse health outcomes that lead to absenteeism and dropout (Levy, 2017). Furthermore, when sex-specific facilities such as toilets are absent from schools or communities, are located in inconvenient locations, or girls resign to practicing open urination and defecation, they may face increased risks of violence and harassment (Levy, 2017). Violence and harassment not only pose significant threats to physical and psychosocial health but can also impact a girl's dignity, self-esteem, and desire to continue her education. See Sect. 2.1.2.

Not only are female students impacted by this disparity in education facilities, but female teachers face negative consequences to their work as they are limited by the same vulnerabilities in sanitation and hygiene needs created through WASH inequalities.

2.3 Challenge: Reproductive Health

Even with the large reductions in maternal and newborn mortality witnessed over the past decades, there is still an unacceptable number of mothers and infants dying from preventable and treatable conditions, a significant portion being related to a lack of WASH—1 million deaths each year are associated with unclean births (Ali et al., 2006; UNICEF, 2019).

2.3.1 Water Collection During Pregnancy

When venturing to obtain water from a quality source, all women and girls are vulnerable to physical, social, and mental health risks and are exposed to violence and harassment. See Sect. 2.1. When pregnant women have to travel to access water and must carry large loads of water, the consequences can be even more severe for mother and pose significant risks to baby.

The physical demands of walking to collect water have been linked to risks for mother and/or baby including uterine prolapse, abnormal heart rate changes, exhaustion and fatigue, inflammation, nausea, back pain, and hypoxia (Jarski &

Trippett, 1990; SIDA, 2019). They may also be more vulnerable to threats of sexual violence and abuse, which puts women at risk of pregnancy complications such as infectious disease, low birth weight, preterm birth, hypertension, and stillbirth (Lawrence, 2011; WHO, 2021). See Sect. 2.1.2.

2.3.2 Infectious Diseases

Access to adequate WASH programming is essential to providing quality care to reduce infection risks that are a leading cause of morbidity and mortality before, during, and after pregnancy (Ali et al., 2006). While some infectious diseases do not cause serious problems, others pose significant complications and outcomes to mother and baby including low birthweight, preterm birth, miscarriage, birth defects, slow development and growth, hearing and sight loss, sepsis, and even death—infections account for 26% of neonatal deaths and 11% of maternal mortality globally (UNICEF, 2019; WaterAid, 2015; Bhaskar & Chaudhury, 2018).

In many LMICs, even if a woman can access a healthcare facility (HCF) for childbirth, there is a high likelihood that it will not have adequate WASH facilities. According to Holt (2019), in LMICs, 50% of HCFs lack piped on-premises water sources, 33% lack proper sanitation, and 39% lack handwashing soap. However, HCFs are not easily accessible in terms of distance, cost, safety, and sociocultural values and beliefs. Therefore, home births are common, with 78% of all home births occurring in the poorest countries globally (Hernández-Vásquez et al., 2021). Home births face a severe lack of proper WASH practices, with only around 1.5–18% of home births having proper access to safe WASH (Hodin, 2017). Without adequate WASH in HCFs and homes, there is an absence of handwashing, clean birth surfaces and instruments, clean cord cutting, safe water for preparing uncontaminated formula (if needed), and more. All of these shortcomings increase the risks of infectious disease threats and other complications to both mother and baby (Healthy Newborn Network, 2022; Hodin, 2017). While not thoroughly discussed here, all women, but especially those who are pregnant, are at a greater risk of infectious disease exposure due to typical gendered roles of childcare, domestic tasks like cooking and cleaning, and agricultural work.

3 Gender-Transformative Approaches

Eliminating gender inequality and discrimination in WASH exposures and outcomes in all humanitarian contexts will require utilizing an intersectional gender-transformative approach. These approaches aim to transform the harmful gender dynamics that work to construct the discussed challenges (and more) faced by women and girls within and alongside WASH programming and policy (MacArthur et al., 2023). By applying gender-transformative WASH approaches, it is intended to synergistically address social inequalities and to improve WASH outcomes.

Gender-transformative approaches seek to redistribute WASH services, opportunities, responsibilities, resources, power, and leadership more equitably among populations. This is realized through:

- Fostering critical examination of gender inequalities roles, norms, and dynamics.
- Recognizing and strengthening positive gender dynamics.
- Promoting the position of women, girls, and other marginalized groups.
- Identifying and transforming the underlying social structures, policies, and systems that perpetuate and legitimize gender inequalities (Marcus et al., 2022).

While these approaches focus heavily on women and girls, the field must continue to integrate other marginalized groups and diversities into planning and policy, utilizing an intersectional-transformative approach that eliminates WASH discrimination and inequalities for all (MacArthur et al., 2023).

Table 1 synthesizes actions proposed across the current literature to achieve a gender-transformative objective.

4 Moving Forward—Women and Gender in Humanitarian Sector Leadership

While gender-transformative approaches to WASH challenges are conceptualized, there is a lack of actualization among programming and policy. While there are many barriers, the absent capacity of the humanitarian system to, itself, be diverse, accountable, and gender-inclusive at all levels is regarded in the literature as a leading cause for this lack of actualization.

While women and girls in target populations are disproportionately burdened and women account for almost half of field staff working among these populations, there is an underrepresentation of women humanitarian leaders among non-governmental aid agencies, governmental agencies, academia, and within the global health community (Patel et al., 2020). Women are assessed to have different leadership styles compared to men, generally focusing on transformational, democratic approaches. Combining these styles with their greater ability to connect with and understand the perspectives and needs of women and girls, women's representation in leadership in the humanitarian system would allow for experience-based representation, empathy, and the push for gender-transformative approaches to come to the forefront (Patel et al., 2020). Furthermore, to ensure the humanitarian system fully takes up the marker of gender-transformation, it is recommended that the humanitarian sector/organizations invest in the capacity and inclusion of gender experts and women's rights/empowerment organizations (Oxfam, 2013). Such persons and groups have specified, focused knowledge and work related to practicing, strengthening, and leveraging gender-sensitive and gender-responsive policies, assessments, practices, standards, and indicators. As many women's organizations and grass-roots movements are women-led, liaisons with such groups

Table 1 Gender-transformative WASH approaches

Program area	Design and methods
Improve the collection and analysis of disaggregated WASH data, especially by sex and gender	Mainstream gender and sex as disaggregated markers of WASH needs and progress (SIDA, 2019) Perform sex and gender data disaggregation by stages across the life course (such as pregnancy and menopause) (Kayser, 2019) Aim to achieve global standards for the collection and monitoring of gender-responsive data (Dickin & Gabrielsson, 2023) Expand WASH indicators beyond access and household infrastructure measures—characterize indicators aligning with gender-specific topics such as decision-making power, risk of violence, school absenteeism/dropout, menstrual hygiene, and more (Dickin & Gabrielsson, 2023)
Collect baseline quantitative and qualitative data to understand the pre-existing gender constructs and the impact of these on systemic inequalities, vulnerabilities, and oppression in WASH	Collect quantitative and qualitative individual, household, and community-level data through improved surveys and interviews directed toward women and girls (Government of Canada, 2019) Perform contextual gender analyses in communities where WASH interventions are being planned to understand the gender realities and requirements of the target population (Water Aid, 2022) Integrate women and girls and trusted community leaders into the conduction of data collection and analysis, and program monitoring and evaluation (UNICEF, 2017)
Develop and establish priority metrics and indicators for monitoring gender topics in WASH	Incorporate gender equality and social inclusion (GESI) indicators into WASH monitoring and evaluation (Carrard et al., 2022) Develop individual-level metrics and tools for WASH data collection, to add to household and community-level metrics (Dickin & Gabrielsson, 2023)
Improve data sharing and communication of WASH inequalities	Enhance open data practices on current WASH data platforms to provide downloadable datasets and data visualizations (Dickin & Gabrielsson, 2023)

(continued)

Table 1 (continued)

Program area	Design and methods
Ensure the equitable role of women and girls in the planning, implementation, management, and evaluation and monitoring of WASH programming and policy	Engage women directly in WASH problem-solving and decision-making in their communities, with local government, and with aid groups (Oxfam, 2019) Provide general literacy, health literacy, public speaking, and communication skill learning opportunities for women to ensure their meaningful participation on committees and governing bodies (Inter-Agency Standing Committee, 2018) Provide targeted training to women and girls on their rights regarding WASH (Oxfam, 2022) Qualitatively and quantitatively monitor and evaluate the participation of women on WASH committees and governing bodies (Inter-Agency Standing Committee, 2018) The involvement of women in WASH programming may increase their workload and responsibilities or they may face negative attitudes from culturally stringent community members—reduce these burdens, by providing support to women and girls engaged in WASH decision-making and leadership. This can include childcare services during participation, the provision of soap or other basic hygiene materials for the home, cash-assistance, and others (UN Women, 2018) Introduce mandatory quotas (for women) on local and national WASH committees and governing bodies (Oxfam, 2022)

(continued)

Table 1 (continued)

Program area	Design and methods
Seek the engagement of men and boys in WASH and gender topics	Work with men and trusted community leaders to sensitize them to the need and benefits of women's and girls' equal participation in decision-making and action planning (Water Aid, 2022) Support and encourage men and boys to take more active roles in caregiving, domestic work, and community WASH actions. This includes providing them with knowledge and information about the rights of women and utilizing trusted community leaders to promote gender equality in local organizations (Oxfam, 2013) Conduct contextual assessments to understand the barriers and attitudes of men and boys towards their own engagement in unpaid domestic work (Oxfam, 2022)
Develop WASH-related enterprise opportunities, especially for women	Institute income generation roles for women within WASH (MacArthur et al., 2023) Identify barriers at the household, community, and institutional levels faced by women to participate in the paid public sphere (Carrard et al., 2022)

can deliver the necessary guidance, accountability, and capacity to ensure the necessary promotion of women's leadership in the humanitarian sector (Oxfam, 2019).

By promoting female leaders and utilizing the capacity and expertise of women's rights/empowerment organizations, WASH assessments and responding programming and policy systems can be strengthened through gender-transformative approaches to reduce disparities and vulnerabilities and promote resiliency, dignity, and power of women and girls in all aspects of their lives.

References

Ali, T., Fikree, F., Rahbar, M., & Mahmud, S. (2006). Frequency and determinants of vaginal infection in postpartum period: A cross-sectional survey from low socioeconomic settlements Karachi, Pakistan. *The Journal of the Pakistan Medical Association, 56*, 99–103.

Bhaskar, A., & Chaudhury, K. (2018). Drinking water contaminants: Maternal and fetal health risks. *Indian Institute of Technology Kharagpur.* https://docs.lib.purdue.edu/cgi/viewcontent.cgi?article=1015&context=swadin

Carrard, N., MacArthur, J., Leahy, C., Soeters, S., & Willetts, J. (2022). The water, sanitation and hygiene gender equality measure (WASH-GEM): Conceptual foundations and domains of change. *Womens Studies International Forum, 91*, 102563. https://doi.org/10.1016/j.wsif.2022.102563

Caruso, B. A., Clasen, F., Hadley, C., Yount, K. M., Haardörfer, R., Rout, M., Dasmohapatra, M., & Cooper, H. L. F. (2017). Understanding and defining sanitation insecurity: Women's gendered experiences of urination, defecation and menstruation in rural Odisha India. *BMJ Global Health, 2*(4), 1–12.

Centers for Disease Control and Prevention. (2022). *Global water, sanitation, and hygiene (WASH).* U.S. Department of Health and Human Services. https://www.cdc.gov/healthywater/global/index.html

Dickin, S., & Gabrielsson, S. (2023). Inequalities in water, sanitation and hygiene: Challenges and opportunities for measurement and monitoring. *Water Security, 20*(6), 100143. https://doi.org/10.1016/j.wasec.2023.100143

Government of Canada. (2019). *Feminist approach—Innovation and effectiveness guidance note.* https://www.international.gc.ca/world-monde/issues_development-enjeux_developpement/priorities-priorites/fiap_ie-paif_ie.aspx?lang=eng

Healthy Newborn Network. (2022). *Newborn health in emergencies.* https://www.healthynewbornnetwork.org/issue/emergencies/

Hernández-Vásquez, A., Chacón-Torrico, H., & Bendezu-Quispe, G. (2021). Prevalence of home birth among 880,345 women in 67 low- and middle-income countries: A meta-analysis of demographic and health surveys. *SSM Population Health, 16*, 100955. https://doi.org/10.1016/j.ssmph.2021.100955

Hirve, S., Lele, P., Sundaram, N., Chavan, U., Weiss, M., Steinmann, P., & Juvekar, S. (2015). Psychosocial stress associated with sanitation practices: Experiences of women in a rural community in India. *Journal of Water.* https://doi.org/10.2166/washdev.2014.110

Hodin, S. (2017, March 22). Giving birth without clean water. Maternal health task force. *Harvard Chan School.*

Holt, K. (2019). Water, sanitation, and hygiene. *Maternal Child Survival Programme.* https://www.mcsprogram.org/our-work/water-sanitation-hygiene-wash/

Human Rights Watch. (2017, April 9). *Going to the toilet when you want.* https://www.hrw.org/report/2017/04/19/going-toilet-when-you-want/sanitation-human-right

Inter-Agency Standing Committee. (2018). *How to support survivors of gender-based violence when a GBV actor is not available in your area: A step-by-step pocket guide for humanitarian practitioners—Version 2.0.* United Nations. https://gbvguidelines.org/wp/wp-content/uploads/2018/03/GBV_Background_Note021718.pdf

Jalali, R. (2021). The role of water, sanitation, hygiene, and gender norms on women's health: A conceptual framework. *Gendered Perspectives on International Development, 1*, 21–44. https://doi.org/10.1353/gpi.2021.0001

Jarski, R. W., & Trippett, D. L. (1990). The risks and benefits of exercise during pregnancy. *Journal of Family Practice, 30*(2), 185–189.

Kayser, G. L., Rao, N., Jose, R., & Raj, A. (2019). Water, sanitation and hygiene: Measuring gender equality and empowerment. *Bulletin of the World Health Organization, 97*(6), 438–440. https://doi.org/10.2471/BLT.18.223305

Kimutai, J. J., Lund, C., Moturi, W. N., Shewangizaw, S., Feyasa, M., & Hanlon, C. (2023). Evidence on the links between water insecurity, inadequate sanitation and mental health: A systematic review and meta-analysis. *PLoS ONE.* https://doi.org/10.1371/journal.pone.0286146

Lawrence, R. M. (2011). Transmission of infectious diseases through breast milk and breastfeeding. *Breastfeeding.* https://doi.org/10.1016/B978-1-4377-0788-5.10013-6

Levy, J. K. (2017, February 13). *Gender, education, and global health: What's the big deal about toilets?.* Washington University of St. Louis, Institute for Public Health. https://publichealth.wustl.edu/gender-education-global-health-whats-big-deal-toilets/#:~:text=When%20a%20girl%20reaches%20puberty,if%20they%20are%20using%20them

MacArthur, J., Carrar, N., Mott, J., Raetz, S., Siscawati, M., & Willetts, J. (2023). Gender equality approaches in water, sanitation, and hygiene programs: Towards gender-transformative practice. *Frontiers.* https://doi.org/10.3389/frwa.2023.1090002

Marcus, R., Samuels, F., Jalal, S., & Belachew, H. (2022). *Gender-transformative programming.* United Nations Children's Fund. https://www.unicef.org/lac/en/media/43146/file

McMichael, C. (2019). Water, sanitation, and hygiene (WASH) in schools in low-income countries: A review of evidence of impact. *International Journal of Environmental Research and Public Health, 16*(3), 359. https://doi.org/10.3390/ijerph16030359

Office for the Coordination of Humanitarian Affairs. (2017, March 2). *WASH interventions in disease outbreak response.* United Nations. https://reliefweb.int/report/world/wash-interventions-disease-outbreakresponse#:~:text=What%20are%20water%2C%20sanitation%20and,in%20a%20variety%20of%20settings

Oxfam. (2013). *Gender issues in conflict and humanitarian action.* https://policy-practice.oxfam.org/resources/gender-issues-in-conflict-and-humanitarian-action-305870/

Oxfam. (2019). *Gender and water, sanitation, and hygiene.*https://doi.org/10.1080/13552074.2017.1349867

Oxfam. (2022, March). *Achieving sustainable development goals 5 and 6.* https://oxfamilibrary.openrepository.com/bitstream/handle/10546/620967/bn-achieving-sdgs-5-6-gender-water-220320-en.pdf?sequence=1

Patel, P., Meagher, K., El Achi, N., Ekzayez, A., Sullivan, R., & Bowsher, G. (2020). Having more women humanitarian leaders will help transform the humanitarian system: Challenges and opportunities for women leaders in conflict and humanitarian health. *Conflict and Health, 14*, 84. https://doi.org/10.1186/s13031-020-00330-9

Routray, P., Schmidt, W. P., Boisson, S., Clasen, T., & Jenkins, M. W. (2015). Socio-cultural and behavioural factors constraining latrine adoption in rural coastal Odisha: An exploratory qualitative study. *BMC Public Health, 15*, 880. https://doi.org/10.1186/s12889-015-2206-3

Sahoo, K. C., Hulland, K. R. S., Caruso, B. A., Swain, R., Freeman, M. C., Panigrahi, P., & Dreibelbis, R. (2015). Sanitation-related psychosocial stress: A grounded theory study of women across the life-course in Odisha, India. *Social Science and Medicine, 139*, 80–89.

Sommer, M., Ferron, S., Cavill, S., & House, S. (2014). Violence, gender, and WASH: Spurring action on a complex, under-documented and sensitive topic. *Environment and Urbanization.* https://doi.org/10.1177/0956247814564528

Sultana, F., & Crow, B. (2000). Water concerns in rural Bangladesh: A gendered perspective. *Pickford J WEDC Conference,* 416–419.

Swedish International Development Cooperation Agency. (2019, August 12). *Gender equality and water, sanitation, and hygiene.* https://www.sida.se/en/publications/gender-equality-and-water-sanitation-and-hygiene

Tallma, P. S., Collins, S., Salmon-Mulanovich, G., Rusyidi, B., Kothadia, A., & Cole, S. (2022). Water insecurity and gender-based violence: A global review of the evidence. *Wiley Interdisciplinary Reviews, 10*(1), e1619. https://doi.org/10.1002/wat2.1619

U.S. Department of Health and Human Services. (2021, March 1). *Effects of violence against women.* https://www.womenshealth.gov/relationships-and-safety/effects-violence-against-women

United Nations Development Programme. (2006). *Human development report 2006.*https://hdr.undp.org/en/content/human-development-report-2006

United Nations Development Programme. (2010, October). Gender and disasters. *Bureau for Crisis Prevention and Recovery.* New York, NY.

United Nations Children's Fund. (2015, February 28). *Advancing WASH in schools monitoring, 2015.* https://reliefweb.int/report/world/advancing-wash-schools-monitoring-2015

United Nations Children's Fund (2016a). *UNICEF: Collecting water is often a colossal waste of time for women and girls.* https://www.unicef.org/press-releases/unicef-collecting-water-often-colossal-waste-time-women-and-girls

United Nations Children's Fund. (2016b). *Water, sanitation and hygiene (WASH).* https://www.unicef.org/wash

United Nations Children's Fund. (2017). *Annual results report 2017: Gender equality.* https://www.unicef.org/media/47776/file/Annual_Results_Report_2017_Gender_Equality.pdf

United Nations Women. (2018). *Gender equality in the 2030 agenda: Gender-responsive water and sanitation systems.* https://www.unwomen.org/sites/default/files/Headquarters/Attachments/

Sections/Library/Publications/2018/Issue-brief-Gender-responsive-water-and-sanitation-systems-en.pdf
United Nations Children's Fund. (2019). *Guidance on menstrual health and hygiene.* https://www.unicef.org/media/91341/file/UNICEF-Guidance-menstrual-health-hygiene-2019.pdf
United Nations. (2024). *SDG goals: Clean water and sanitation.* https://unstats.un.org/sdgs/report/2023/Goal-06/#:~:text=However%2C%20in%202022%2C%202.2%20billion,with%20soap%20and%20water%20at
Water Aid. (2022). *Integrating gender equality into water, sanitation and hygiene projects.* https://washmatters.wateraid.org/sites/g/files/jkxoof256/files/integrating-gender-equality-into-water-sanitation-and-hygiene-projects-guidance-for-ngos-and-implementing-partners.pdf
WaterAid. (2015). A*nnual report and financial statements: 2014–2015.* https://www.wateraid.org/uk/sites/g/files/jkxoof211/files/wateraid-annual-report-2014-15.pdf
World Health Organization. (2019). *Burden of disease attributable to unsafe drinking-water, sanitation and hygiene.* United Nations. https://iris.who.int/bitstream/handle/10665/370026/9789240075610-eng.pdf?sequence=1&isAllowed=y
World Health Organization. (2021, March 9). *Violence against women prevalence estimates, 2018.* United Nations. https://www.who.int/publications/i/item/9789240022256
World Health Organization. (2023, July 6). *Women and girls bear brunt of water and sanitation crisis—new UNICEF-WHO report.* United Nations.https://www.who.int/news/item/06-07-2023-women-and-girls-bear-brunt-of-water-and-sanitation-crisis-new-unicef-who-report

7 Determinants of Sexual and Gender-Based Violence Against Refugee Women and Girls

Kelly E. Fraser

Abstract

Refugee women and girls of all ages face a high prevalence of sexual and gender-based violence (SGBV), which is associated with negative mental and physical health outcomes. This paper seeks to identify the determinants for female refugees' experience of SGBV as well as their ability to seek care after being abused. A search of the available literature located 26 articles which addressed SGBV determinants for refugee women and girls. The review of the literature revealed eight categories of risk for experiencing SGBV: migration and displacement, economic vulnerability, cultural attitudes, marriage, substance abuse, social support, prior history of abuse, and the COVID-19 pandemic. Six categories of determinants were found for female refugees' access to care services: awareness of services and rights, legal status in the host community, trust in healthcare providers, social barriers, security, and the COVID-19 pandemic. Interventions to prevent SGBV against refugee women and girls should focus on the migration process, cultural attitudes toward gender roles, pre-existing vulnerabilities in the refugee population, and the impact of interventions for other public health issues. Further research is needed to build an evidence base for interventions in these four areas.

Keywords

Refugees • Sexual and gender-based violence • Women • Girls • Determinants

K. E. Fraser (✉)
College of Public Health, University of South Florida, 13201 Bruce B. Downs Blvd, MDC 56, Tampa, FL 33612, USA

S. Spowart (ed.), *Global Happiness and Humanitarian Assistance*, Integrated Science 29, https://doi.org/10.1007/978-3-031-71789-5_7

1 Determinants of Sexual and Gender-Based Violence Against Refugee Women and Girls

At the end of 2022, there were more than 35.3 million refugees and asylum seekers globally, more than half of whom are women and girls (United Nations High Commissioner for Refugees (UNHCR, 2023a; UNHCR, 2023b). This population is growing steadily; from 2012 through 2022, there was a more than 3.5-fold increase in the total number of female refugees (UNHCR, 2023b). Ongoing conflicts and other humanitarian emergencies in the Democratic Republic of the Congo, Sudan, Myanmar, Somalia, and elsewhere are expected to continue to force populations from their homes and across borders through 2023 and beyond (UNHCR, 2023a).

Gender-based violence (GBV)—also referred to as sexual and gender-based violence (SBGV)—is defined by the United Nations Inter-Agency Standing Committee (IASC) and UNHCR as "an umbrella term for any harmful act that is perpetrated against a person's will and that is based on socially ascribed (i.e. gender) differences between males and females" (IASC, 2015; UNHCR, 2020). This term encompasses a wide range of harmful practices, including physical, verbal, emotional, and sexual abuse; intimate partner violence (IPV), sexual harassment, sexual assault, and rape; sexual coercion, forced prostitution, and human trafficking; female genital mutilation (FGM); and forced marriage, including child marriage (IASC, 2015; UNHCR, 2020). Men, women, boys, and girls can all be subjected to gender-based violence; however, women and girls are at a higher risk (IASC, 2015; UNHCR, 2020).

Refugee women and girls of all ages face high prevalence of sexual and gender-based violence in a wide range of settings (Delkhosh et al., 2019; Islam et al., 2022; Kong et al., 2023; Logie et al., 2019; Mezzatesta Gava et al., 2022; Odwe et al., 2018; Um et al., 2018). In a cross—sectional survey of Afghan women refugees in Iran, 80% reported experiencing IPV in the past year (Delkhosh et al., 2019). A separate study found a similar prevalence among female refugees and asylum seekers in Montreal, Canada: 80% of such women reported experiencing gender—based violence, including two-thirds of women who were claiming asylum for unrelated reasons (Mezzatesta Gava et al., 2022). Among Rohingya refugee women surveyed in 2022, 72% reported being hit or beaten by husband and 57% reported being forced to have sex in last 12 months (Islam et al., 2022). In a survey of adult Congolese women seeking asylum in Uganda, 80% of refugees reported being raped at least once, with 55% experiencing multiple rapes (Familiar et al., 2021).

Young women and girls are also vulnerable to SGBV (Kong et al., 2023; Logie et al., 2019). A cross-sectional survey of young adult women ages 16–24 in informal refugee settlements in Uganda found that more than 50% had experienced violence as young adults, and that almost 10% had experienced multiple forms of violence (Logie et al., 2019). Similarly, in the Kule refugee camp in Ethiopia, a cross sectional survey of female students in 5th through 8th grade—two-thirds of whom were teenagers—found that nearly 35% had been raped (Kong et al., 2023).

Many refugee women are subjected to multiple forms of sexual and gender-based violence (Odwe et al., 2018; Um et al., 2018). In a survey of female heads of household in the Rwamwanja refugee camp in Uganda, 72% of women reported experiencing some form of SGBV; of these, nearly 70% of women reported physical abuse and 63% reported sexual abuse from a partner (Odwe et al., 2018). Another survey of North Korean women refugees in South Korea found that 43.9% had experienced two or more forms of abuse—either physical, emotional, sexual, or economic (Um et al., 2018). Similarly, Hossain et al. (2020) found that of the women in the Dadaab refugee camps in Kenya who experienced intimate partner violence, 63% were subjected to multiple forms of abuse.

2 Problem

Gender-based violence has been linked to a range of negative physical health outcomes (Baranowski et al., 2019; Familiar et al., 2021; Kong et al., 2023; Rometsch et al., 2020; Wachter et al., 2018; Wikholm et al., 2020). A cross-sectional survey of Yazidi refugee women who fled to Germany after being victimized by the Islamic State reported pain, shortness of breath, and difficulty walking; these symptoms were attributed to both physical and psychological causes (Rometsch et al., 2020). Health records from Central American asylum seekers showed that more than a third of women evaluated reported lacerations or blunt trauma to the head or body as a result of GBV (Baranowski et al., 2019).

Victims of sexual violence also reported physical injuries and other health consequences (Familiar et al., 2021; Kong et al., 2023; Wikholm et al., 2020). A cross-sectional survey of Congolese refugees in Uganda reported that 87% of women who were raped experienced injuries as a result of the assault, and more than a quarter became pregnant (Familiar et al., 2021). In a study of female asylum-seekers in the United States who reported experiencing female genital mutilation (FGM), more than three quarters reported acute bleeding and difficulty with intercourse, and more than half experienced pregnancy complications (Wikholm et al., 2020). While rates of sexually-transmitted infections have not been assessed, Kong et al. (2023) found that 80% of students surveyed in the Kule refugee camp who had been raped indicated that the perpetrator did not use a condom, putting them at higher risk for both HIV and other STIs.

Refugee women exposed to gender-based violence also have a high risk of poor mental health outcomes including depression, anxiety, and post-traumatic stress disorder (PTSD) (Baranowski et al., 2019; Familiar et al., 2021; Hossain et al., 2020; Laughon et al., 2023; Lever et al., 2019; Nam et al., 2022a; Pérez-Vázquez & Bonilla-Campos, 2023; Um et al., 2021; Wikholm et al., 2020). Studies of refugee women in a variety of settings found rates of depression ranging from 36 to 100%, anxiety ranging from 41 to 92%, and PSTD ranging from 50 to 80% (Baranowski et al., 2019; Familiar et al., 2021; Hossain et al., 2020; Lever et al., 2019; Wikholm et al., 2020). In a cross-sectional survey of Congolese refugees in Uganda, Familiar et al. (2021) found that being raped more than doubled the odds of experiencing

PTSD and depression. Suicide risks were also high among refugee women who experienced SGBV (Nam et al., 2022a; Um et al., 2021). In separate surveys of North Korean women refugees in South Korea, Um et al. (2021) found that 54% of those who had experienced sexual violence before migration were at risk of suicide, while Nam et al. (2022a) reported that women who experienced gender-based violence were 16 times more likely to attempt suicide.

Given the increasing numbers of refugees across the world each year, the high prevalence of SGBV among refugee women and girls, and the seriousness of mental and physical health outcomes among survivors of sexual and gender-based violence, it is clear that SGBV will continue to pose a significant public health problem for this population. It is crucial for states that host refugee populations, organizations that serve refugees, and the public health community to be aware of the factors that may impact the likelihood of refugee woman and girls experiencing SGBV and their ability to seek support after being victimized, so they can identify opportunities and priorities for interventions. This literature review therefore seeks to outline the determinants for refugee women and girls' experiences of SGBV, as well as their access to care.

3 Data Sources and Methods

A literature review was conducted via PubMed using the following key words: "gender—based violence", "sexual violence", "GBV", "SGBV", "rape", "women", "girls", and "refugees", resulting in an initial set of n = 371 articles. Articles were excluded if they were published before 2018, were not available in English, did not address sexual and gender-based violence, focused solely or primarily on male victims, or focused on non-refugee populations such as internally displaced persons or host communities. Remaining articles were included only if they addressed determinants for experiencing sexual and gender-based violence or for care seeking behavior among SGBV victims. After applying inclusion and exclusion criteria, a final sample of n = 26 articles were selected for this analysis.

4 Results

The review of the literature revealed eight categories of determinants for refugee women and girls' experience of SGBV: migration and displacement, economic vulnerability, cultural attitudes, marriage, substance abuse, social support, prior history of abuse, and the COVID-19 pandemic. Six categories of determinants were found for female refugees' access to care services: awareness of services and rights, legal status in the host community, trust in healthcare providers, social barriers, security, and the COVID-19 pandemic.

4.1 Risk and Protective Factors for Experiencing SGBV

4.1.1 Migration and Displacement

Women and girls are at a heightened risk for gender-based violence during the migration process (Baranowski et al., 2019; Gebreyesus et al., 2019; Kim et al., 2022; Laughon et al., 2023). Baranowski et al. (2019) found that more than a third of women who received psychological evaluations after traveling from Honduras, El Salvador, and Guatemala to the United States reported experiencing violence at some point during their journey. Victimization can happen at any point in the refugees' journey; in a series of focus group discussions with Eritrean refugees who fled to Israel, Gebreyesus et al. (2019) noted that the women experienced SGBV upon leaving their home countries, while transiting through the region, and near the border of their destination country.

Dependence on human smugglers—typically men—to assist with crossing borders can expose women to sexual assault, kidnappings for ransom, and human trafficking (Baranowski et al., 2019; Gebreyesus et al., 2019). Women may also be targeted by gangs, bandits, and other migrants during their journey (Baranowski et al., 2019; Gebreyesus et al., 2018, 2019; Kim et al., 2022; Laughon et al., 2023). Even exposure to violence against other women can traumatize refugees; in interviews with female asylum seekers in an informal encampment on the U.S.-Mexico border, Laughon et al. (2023) reported that many women were in a state of constant vigilance after witnessing attacks against other migrants during their journey and in the camp and from hearing rumors about attacks against children.

4.1.2 Economic Vulnerability

Upon arrival to the host country, many refugees are unable to work due to restrictive laws in the host country or a lack of opportunities in camp settings (Gebreyesus et al., 2018; Sharma et al., 2020a; Wachter et al., 2018). Men's inability to work and provide for their families can create tension at home and serve as a driver for violent behaviors against women, particularly their wives (Fry et al., 2019; Gebreyesus et al., 2018; Wachter et al., 2018). In focus group discussions held by Gebreyesus et al. (2018) with Ethiopian asylum-seekers in Israel and by Wachter et al. (2018) with refugees in camp settings in South Sudan, Kenya, and Iraq, both men and women identified arguments about financial issues as precursors to intimate partner violence.

A lack of educational opportunities for women can also make them more vulnerable to abuse (Baranowski et al., 2019; Roupetz et al., 2020; Sharma et al., 2020a; Wringe et al., 2019). In a survey of female headed households in the Rwamwanja refugee settlement in Uganda, 69% of women reported having no formal education at all (Odwe et al., 2018). In a review of records from female asylum seekers from Central America, Baranowski et al., 2019 noted that 63% had been forced to drop out of school earlier in life, most often to support their families. Similar patterns have been noted in camp settings, in which refugee girls are forced to abandon their studies to get married, to avoid sexual harassment, or as a result of being raped (Kong et al., 2023; Roupetz et al., 2020; Sharma et al., 2020a; Wringe et al., 2019).

This lack of formal status and education forces female refugees to turn to the informal sector for work (Gebreyesus et al., 2018; Roupetz et al., 2020; Wachter et al., 2018). However, even when women are able to find employment, they may face sexual harassment while working or traveling to work (Gebreyesus et al., 2018; Wachter et al., 2018). Some women turn to prostitution or are sexually exploited by their employers in other sectors (Gebreyesus et al., 2018; Roupetz et al., 2020). Lack of formal protections for refugee workers in the host community and a lack of security in camp settings leave women vulnerable to continued abuse (Gebreyesus et al., 2018; Roupetz et al., 2020). Women who earn money outside the home may also be subject to financial abuse from intimate partners who confiscate their earnings (Wachter et al., 2018).

4.1.3 Cultural Attitudes

Cultural attitudes toward traditional gender roles were identified as a risk factor for gender-based violence in several studies (Bermudez et al., 2019; Fry et al., 2019; Odwe et al., 2018; Pérez-Vázquez & Bonilla-Campos, 2023; Sharma et al., 2020a; Um et al., 2018; Wachter et al., 2018). Fry et al. (2019) found that male socialization creates cultural expectations for men to assert power and control, pursue sexual conquests, and act aggressively; while refugee men whose masculinity is threatened by a loss of power and control may lash out violently through GBV. In focus group discussions with refugees living in camps in Ethiopia, South Sudan, Kenya, and Iraq, participants described cultural expectations that women behave submissively and be subservient to their husbands, that men should hold all decision-making power in society, and that men have ownership over their wives (Sharma et al., 2020a; Wachter et al., 2018).

These attitudes translated into societal support for intimate partner violence, as both men and women indicated support for husbands beating their wives in some circumstances (Islam et al., 2022; Odwe et al., 2018; Sharma et al., 2020a; Wachter et al., 2018). In a cross-sectional survey of refugees in the Rwamwanja camp in Uganda, women actually expressed greater belief that IPV was justifiable if men were angry at their partners than men did, with 56% of women expressing support compared to 20% of men (Odwe et al., 2018). A similar phenomenon was described by Islam et al. (2022), who found that 87% of Rohingya refugee women surveyed believed beatings were justified if women argued with their husbands.

Internalized support for gender-based violence was also found to be a risk factor for actually experiencing abuse (Bermudez et al., 2019; Um et al., 2018). In a survey of North Korean refugees living in South Korea, Um et al. (2018) found that support for traditional gender roles more than doubled the odds of having experienced physical abuse in the past year. In a survey of teenage girls in refugee camps in Ethiopia, those who accepted norms of gender inequality were more likely to experience rape or transactional sex (Bermudez et al., 2019).

4.1.4 Marriage

Multiple studies found that refugee women and girls were at risk of forced marriage and child marriage (El Arab & Sagbakken, 2019; Gebreyesus et al., 2019; Roupetz et al., 2020; Sharma et al., 2020a; Wachter et al., 2018; Wringe et al., 2019). While Gebreyesus et al. (2019) and Kim et al. (2022) noted instances of women being kidnapped and forced to marry their captors during their migration journeys, most studies discussed forced marriages that took place after resettlement, usually at the family's behest. In some settings, marriage is perceived by adults as a protective factor for young women against experiencing sexual harassment, assault, and economic hardship (El Arab & Sagbakken, 2019; Roupetz et al., 2020; Wringe et al., 2019). Therefore, a lack of economic and physical security may serve as risk factors for increased rates of forced marriage and child marriage. Societal norms promoting early marriage and social stigma against unmarried women also serve as drivers for forced and child marriage in some contexts (El Arab & Sagbakken, 2019; Roupetz et al., 2020; Sharma et al., 2020a).

On the other hand, Sharma et al. (2020a) found that rates of forced marriage and child marriage were lower among Somali refugees in the Bokolmayo refugee camp in Ethiopia than in their home communities in Somalia. In focus groups, refugees identified access to education, physical security in the camps, and reduced social stigma against unmarried women over the age of 21 as protective factors against child marriages (Sharma et al., 2020a). Unlike other studies which found economic hardship to be a driver of forced marriages, in this setting it was also protective as it reduced men's ability to pay a substantial dowry, thereby lowering the financial incentives for parents to marry off their daughters (Sharma et al., 2020a). Ethiopian laws against child marriage and polygamy, as well as awareness programs from NGOs discouraging marriage before the age of 18, were also identified as important factors in reducing the rates of child marriage (Sharma et al., 2020a).

Several studies found cultural beliefs that women did not have the right to refuse sex in the context of marriage (Islam et al., 2022; Sharma et al., 2020a; Wachter et al., 2018). In focus group discussions, some refugees indicated that marital rape and intimate partner violence were at least somewhat justified if a women refused to have sex with her husband (Sharma et al., 2020a; Wachter et al., 2018). In their survey of Rohingya refugee women, Islam et al. (2022), 68% believed they could not refuse to have sex with their husband, and this belief had a statistically significant association with women's belief that beatings could be justified.

Marriage itself was also found to be a source of intimate partner violence (IPV), a form of gender-based violence (Logie et al., 2019; Roupetz et al., 2020; Sharma et al., 2020a; Wachter et al., 2018; Wringe et al., 2019). Logie et al. (2019) found that young married women had three times higher odds of experiencing intimate partner violence than their unmarried peers. Multiple studies found that strong support for traditional gender roles served as a risk factor for cultural acceptance of IPV in the context of marriage and perpetuated the belief that women shared the blame for instances of IPV (Pérez-Vázquez & Bonilla-Campos, 2023; Roupetz et al., 2020; Sharma et al., 2020a; Wachter et al., 2018). In camp settings, increased freedom for women and girls was perceived by men as threatening to their role in society and marriage (Sharma et al., 2020a; Wachter et al., 2018). In focus group discussions with refugees in camps in South Sudan, Kenya, and Iraq, Wachter et al. (2018) reported that many respondents identified upended gender roles, women acting less submissively, and men's inability to serve as a provider for their families as triggers for physical, emotional, verbal, and financial abuse. Attempts to flee abusive marriages can also expose women to further harm, as they may be subjected to social stigma, rejected by their families, or forced to turn to prostitution to support themselves (Roupetz et al., 2020).

4.1.5 Substance Abuse

The use of alcohol, tobacco, and drugs by both female refugees and their partners has been associated with increased risk of sexual and gender-based violence (Kong et al., 2023; Sharma et al., 2020b; Wachter et al., 2018). In East Africa, multiple studies have identified the use of khat, a locally available stimulant, by both men and women as a risk factor for intimate partner violence (Kong et al., 2023; Sharma et al., 2020b; Wachter et al., 2018). In focus group discussions with refugees in camp settings, community members identified social pressures to engage in substance abuse, the stress of living in camps, and unemployment as drivers for men to abuse alcohol and drugs (Sharma et al., 2020b; Wachter et al., 2018). Alcohol was identified as a cause of violent behavior, while long-term khat use was associated with social withdrawal, anger, and physical and sexual aggression (Sharma et al., 2020b; Wachter et al., 2018). Refugees also reported that men diverting household funds to spend on drugs and alcohol created tension in the family and can lead to IPV (Sharma et al., 2020b; Wachter et al., 2018). While less common, women's substance use was also associated with increased odds of victimization; in a cross-sectional survey of refugee girls attending elementary school in Kule refugee camp, girls who smoked had four times higher odds of being raped and girls who drank alcohol had three times higher odds of being raped (Kong et al., 2023).

4.1.6 Social Support

Social support at the interpersonal and community levels serves as a protective factor against sexual and gender-based violence (Odwe et al., 2018; Treves-Kagan et al., 2022; Um et al., 2021; Wachter et al., 2018). Wachter et al. (2018) described support from parents and families as protective factors against abuse, as is the presence of the husband's family to observe his behavior and intervene when needed. On the other hand, separation from family due to displacement is a risk factor for IPV, and the husband's family can also act as a driver for violence if his parents dislike his wife (Wachter et al., 2018). Social ties can also be protective against negative health outcomes from gender-based violence; a cross-sectional survey of female refugees who fled from North Korea to South Korea found that having strong, diverse social networks and family ties lowered the risk of suicide among victims of sexual assault (Um et al., 2021). At the community level, Odwe et al.

(2018) described perceptions that community does not tolerate GBV as a protective factor encouraging women to seek help. Likewise, data from a randomized controlled trial in refugee-hosting neighborhoods in Ecuador found that neighborhoods that scored higher in measures of social disorganization had higher rates of emotional, physical, and sexual IPV, while social cohesion scores acted as a mediator on the association between social disorganization and emotional IPV (Treves-Kagan et al., 2022). Together, this evidence indicates that supportive family, social, and community ties protect women against gender-based violence and can encourage them to seek help.

4.1.7 Prior History of Abuse

Refugee women who have experienced sexual and gender-based violence in the past, including during childhood, are at an increased risk for experiencing SGBV again (Islam et al., 2022; Logie et al., 2019; Nam et al., 2022b; Um et al., 2018). In one survey of North Korean refugees in South Korea, Nam et al. (2022b) found that women who had been sexually assaulted in their home country were 4.5 times as likely to experience physical abuse after resettlement. Focus group discussions with Rohingya refugees revealed that the reverse was also true: women who had already experienced physical abuse from their husbands were significantly less likely to be able to reject unwanted sexual advances and were therefore more vulnerable to sexual abuse (Islam et al., 2022).

Abuse that occurred years earlier—during childhood—was also a risk factor for SGBV as adults, as one survey of North Korean women refugees in South Korea found that having experienced abuse in childhood more than doubled the odds of experiencing sexual or financial abuse in the past year (Um et al., 2018). Logie et al. (2019) confirmed these findings in a cross–sectional survey of young female refugees in Uganda which found that those who experienced childhood abuse had four times higher odds of experiencing any violence as an adult and five times higher odds of experiencing multiple forms of violence.

4.1.8 COVID-19 Pandemic

Two studies addressed increased vulnerability to gender-based violence among refugee women and girls during the COVID-19 pandemic (Gillespie et al., 2022; Phillimore et al., 2022). In a survey of refugee GBV survivors and services providers in several countries, Phillimore et al. (2022) described how refugees' existing vulnerabilities were exacerbated by the COVID-19 pandemic and its associated lockdowns. Economic stresses were increased due to workplace shutdowns, as refugees were unable to work but were often ineligible for unemployment benefits in their host countries (Phillimore et al., 2022). Many refugees were stuck in overcrowded housing, forcing them to isolate in single rooms or risk exposure to the virus (Phillimore et al., 2022). Support services were reduced and social networks were often inaccessible, especially for poorer refugees who lacked internet access, which left both men and women feeling isolated and hopeless (Gillespie et al., 2022; Phillimore et al., 2022). These factors combined to increase stress at home and raise the risk of intimate partner violence. For women who were subjected to IPV, lockdowns restricted their ability to escape and forced them to spend time isolated with their perpetrators (Gillespie et al., 2022; Phillimore et al., 2022). While the lockdowns associated with the COVID-19 pandemic have ended, future pandemics or other events that isolate refugees and limit their access to services could have similar effects on women's susceptibility to gender-based violence.

4.2 Barriers and Facilitators for Access to SGBV Care

Several studies described a lack of awareness of available services, rights for GBV survivors, and the importance of seeking help as barriers to accessing care for women who have experienced gender-based violence (Muuo et al., 2020; Pérez-Vázquez & Bonilla-Campos, 2023; Rodella Sapia et al., 2020). In a survey of women and aged 18 and up who visited a GBV service center in the Dadaab refugee camp in Kenya, Muuo et al. (2020) found that formal service centers run by NGOs were the most common place for GBV survivors in the camp to seek care, but many women were unaware of the services available to them until they were reached by an awareness campaign. Some victims also minimized the negative impacts of SGBV, which lowered their willingness to seek treatment (Pérez-Vázquez & Bonilla-Campos, 2023). Awareness-raising campaigns about the severity of gender-based violence and the importance of seeking treatment were found to be effective in encouraging women and girls to seek help (Muuo et al., 2020; Pérez-Vázquez & Bonilla-Campos, 2023).

In some contexts, the legal status of refugees in the host country influenced victims' decisions on whether to report their abuse and seek treatment (Pérez-Vázquez & Bonilla-Campos, 2023; Rodella Sapia et al., 2020). In focus group discussions with stakeholders who work with refugees in Switzerland, service providers described how refugees were often reluctant to disclose their experience of GBV due to a lack of confidence in the legal system, particularly if they had negative experiences with authorities or were not protected in transit countries (Rodella Sapia et al., 2020). Refugees whose asylum cases were pending did not always see a benefit to disclosing abuse that occurred in transit or host communities, because only SGBV that occurred in their home countries could assist with their case (Rodella Sapia et al., 2020). In some contexts, the lack of formal status during the asylum process could also restrict victims' access to healthcare services (Rodella Sapia et al., 2020). In cases of intimate partner violence, women reported fears of legal consequences for their husbands that could result in separating their families or restricting their ability to work (Pérez-Vázquez & Bonilla-Campos, 2023).

Refugee women's level of trust in healthcare providers can act as either a barrier or facilitator to seeking GBV-related services (Muuo et al., 2020; Pérez-Vázquez & Bonilla-Campos, 2023; Rodella Sapia et al., 2020). Trust often needs to be built over time, with multiple visits to the same provider before a woman is willing to open up; continuity of care is a crucial facilitator for providers to build these relationships with their patients (Rodella Sapia et al., 2020). Translation services and access to cultural mediators can also facilitate communication between patients and providers and assist with building trust (Pérez-Vázquez & Bonilla-Campos, 2023; Rodella Sapia et al., 2020). Negative interactions with health providers, on the other hand, can damage trust in the healthcare system and discourage women from seeking care (Pérez-Vázquez & Bonilla-Campos, 2023; Rodella Sapia et al., 2020). For example, Rodella Sapia et al. (2020) described cases where women had IUDs inserted without their consent when seeking care in a transit country; when doctors in the host community disclosed the violation, the refugees lost trust in healthcare professionals generally and were reluctant to seek care. Women in both open and camp settings expressed fears that healthcare providers would breach confidentiality, particularly when the service provider is also a member of the refugee community (Muuo et al., 2020; Pérez-Vázquez & Bonilla-Campos, 2023). Disclosures of women's SGBV experiences to her family or community members can make others less likely to seek support (Muuo et al., 2020; Pérez-Vázquez & Bonilla-Campos, 2023).

Social barriers to reporting gender-based violence and seeking care include social stigma, victim blaming, and individual coping strategies (Muuo et al., 2020; Odwe et al., 2018; Pérez-Vázquez & Bonilla-Campos, 2023; Rodella Sapia et al., 2020). Several studies described women's fears of social stigma from their families or communities if others found out they were a victim of GBV or that they were seeking mental health services (Muuo et al., 2020; Pérez-Vázquez & Bonilla-Campos, 2023; Rodella Sapia et al., 2020). In a survey of women in the Rwamwanja refugee camp in Uganda, Odwe et al. (2018) found that women were more likely to support care-seeking if they believed that SGBV was not supported by the community in the camp. On the other hand, women who have the support of their families and social networks may rely on them for support in lieu of seeking formal care services (Rodella Sapia et al., 2020).

Security may also play a role in women's decisions of whether to seek care (Muuo et al., 2020). In cases where the victim knows her attacker, such as her husband or a fellow community member, she may fear future violence or retaliation for making the report, especially if she does not have confidence he will be arrested or removed from the camp (Muuo et al., 2020). In camp settings, security guards may also be a barrier to accessing services; Muuo et al. (2020) found that women in the Dadaab refugee camp in Kenya were denied access to the GBV service center unless they paid bribes to the security guards.

During the COVID-19 pandemic, additional challenges arose that threatened women and girl's access to SGBV services (Gillespie et al., 2022; Phillimore et al., 2022). For women whose abuse was ongoing, many were unable to flee because shelters were not accepting new residents (Phillimore et al., 2022). Many services were cancelled, reduced, or moved online, which proved inaccessible for those without reliable internet access (Gillespie et al., 2022; Phillimore et al., 2022). For those who were able to access healthcare, counseling, or other support services online, the lack of translators or cultural mediators in the new online format created additional communication barriers between refugees and providers (Gillespie et al., 2022). However, women who were able to connect with other refugees often built online communities that provided social solidarity and facilitated their care (Gillespie et al., 2022).

5 Discussion

The results of this literature review revealed intersecting themes for refugee women and girls' vulnerability to experiencing sexual and gender-based violence and for their ability to seek care after being abused. First, the migration process itself requires refugees to flee their homes and travel through often-unsafe transit countries before arriving in their host community. This journey exposes women and girls to vulnerability to exploitation, trafficking, and abuse from human traffickers, gangs, and other migrants (Baranowski et al., 2019; Gebreyesus et al., 2018, 2019; Kim et al., 2022; Laughon et al., 2023). At the same time, a lack of protection by authorities and unethical care from healthcare providers in transit countries may erode their confidence in the health and legal systems, Thus diminishing the likelihood they will seek care even if they eventually arrive in a safe host country (Pérez-Vázquez & Bonilla-Campos, 2023; Rodella Sapia et al., 2020).

Second, restrictions for refugees—and asylum-seekers whose cases are pending—in the host country increases women's economic vulnerability and ability to report abuse. Women and girls who are not authorized to work or attend school may turn to prostitution or informal work, where they are more likely to be abused (Baranowski et al., 2019; Gebreyesus et al., 2018; Roupetz et al., 2020; Sharma et al., 2020a; Wachter et al., 2018; Wringe et al., 2019). At the same time, men's inability to work increases frustration at home and can lead to an increase in intimate partner violence (Fry et al., 2019; Gebreyesus et al., 2018; Wachter et al., 2018). Economic vulnerability also made women more reluctant to report IPV, however, especially if they relied on their husbands financially (Pérez-Vázquez & Bonilla-Campos, 2023).

Third, cultural attitudes related to gender roles, including marriage and the seriousness of gender-based violence, were reflected across multiple categories of determinants. Gender socialization for men and women creates cultural expectations that men should provide for their families and that women should defer to men; when refugees' situations prevent them from fulfilling these roles, men become more likely to lash out through gender-based violence (Fry et al., 2019; Sharma et al., 2020a; Wachter et al., 2018). Cultural expectations for marriage and social stigma against unmarried women contribute to high risks of forced marriage and child marriage, while cultural acceptance of intimate partner violence in the context of marriage lead to high risks for SGBV for married women (El Arab & Sagbakken, 2019; Gebreyesus et al., 2019; Islam et al., 2022; Logie et al., 2019; Odwe et al., 2018; Roupetz et al., 2020; Sharma et al., 2020a; Wachter et al., 2018; Wringe et al., 2019). These cultural expectations can impact how women perceive the seriousness of SGBV and the level of social support women receive from their families and communities, which in turn can impact their likelihood of both experiencing SGBV and seeking care (Muuo et al., 2020; Odwe et al., 2018; Pérez-Vázquez & Bonilla-Campos, 2023; Rodella Sapia et al., 2020; Treves-Kagan et al., 2022; Um et al., 2021; Wachter et al., 2018).

Fourth, refugee women are impacted by other determinants such as substance abuse, prior history of abuse, and awareness of their rights (Islam et al., 2022; Kong et al., 2023; Logie et al., 2019; Nam et al., 2022b; Rodella Sapia et al., 2020; Sharma et al., 2020b; Um et al., 2018; Wachter et al., 2018). While these factors are not unique to their experiences as refugees, they can intersect with and exacerbate other risk factors (e.g., increased economic vulnerability when funds are diverted to purchase drugs or alcohol) (Sharma et al., 2020b; Wachter et al., 2018).

Finally, the COVID-19 pandemic led to lockdowns and interruptions in support services, both of which increased women's vulnerability to abuse and created new barriers to care (Gillespie et al., 2022; Phillimore et al., 2022). While most pandemic-era restrictions have since been lifted, future pandemics or other emergencies could create similar risks for refugee women if policymakers enact such restrictions without safeguards designed with their needs in mind.

5.1 Recommendations

Interventions to prevent, respond to, and treat the effects of sexual and gender-based violence against refugee women and girls should account for the determinants identified in this review. Women and girls traveling through transit countries need access to safe migration routes, reliable and ethical healthcare, and support from local authorities to intervene if they have been victimized. Host communities must ensure refugees have access to employment, education, and information about their legal rights as refugees. SGBV awareness programs must take into account social norms regarding gender roles, marriage, and perceptions of the seriousness of gender-based violence in the community. Interventions for survivors of SGBV should build on existing social networks that serve as protective factors for this community. Prevention efforts should prioritize women and girls with pre-existing vulnerabilities, such as a past history of victimization or substance abuse. Policymakers should also consider the needs of refugee women and girls when designing interventions for other public health problems to avoid unintended consequences that could increase their vulnerability to SGBV or prevent them from seeking help.

5.2 Limitations

This study was affected by the following limitations. The articles included in the literature review used a wide range of methods, including focus group discussions, key informant interviews, cross-sectional surveys, and randomized controlled trials. While this was sufficient for identifying common themes, the variation in study designs made it impractical to make direct comparisons. The use of only one database to locate relevant articles may have introduced selection bias in the literature review. Furthermore, this paper focused only on evidence for determinants of refugee women and girls' experience of SGBV or access to care; it did not review the evidence for effective interventions that address the identified determinants.

6 Conclusion

Refugee women and girls of all ages face a high prevalence of sexual and gender-based violence (SGBV), which is associated with negative mental and physical health outcomes. The literature on SGBV determinants revealed that migration and displacement, economic vulnerability, cultural attitudes, marriage, substance abuse, social support, prior history of abuse, and the COVID-19 pandemic all impacted refugee women and girls' likelihood of experiencing sexual and gender-based violence, while awareness of services and rights, legal status in the host community, trust in healthcare providers, social barriers, security, and the COVID-19 pandemic affected their ability to seek care. These intersecting determinants create opportunities for interventions focused on the migration process, cultural attitudes toward gender roles, pre-existing vulnerabilities in the refugee population, and the impact of interventions for other public health issues, though further research is needed to determine which interventions are most effective for this population.

Acknowledgements This paper has not been previously presented, and there are no conflicts of interest to report.

References

Baranowski, K. A., Wang, E., D'Andrea, M. R., & Singer, E. K. (2019). Experiences of gender-based violence in women asylum seekers from Honduras El Salvador and Guatemala. *Torture, 29*(3), 46–58. https://doi.org/10.7146/torture.v29i3.111970

Bermudez, L. G., Yu, G., Lu, L., Falb, K., Eoomkham, J., Abdella, G., & Stark, L. (2019). HIV risk among displaced adolescent girls in Ethiopia: The role of gender attitudes and self esteem. *Prevention Science, 20*(1), 137–146. https://doi.org/10.1007/s11121-018-0902-9

Delkhosh, M., Merghati Khoei, E., Ardalan, A., Rahimi Foroushani, A., & Gharavi, M. B. (2019). Prevalence of intimate partner violence and reproductive health outcomes among Afghan refugee women in Iran. *Health Care for Women International, 40*(2), 213-237. https://www.doi.org/https://doi.org/10.1080/07399332.2018.1529766

El Arab, R., & Sagbakken, M. (2019). Child marriage of female Syrian refugees in Jordan and Lebanon: A literature review. *Global Health Action, 12*(1), 1585709. https://doi.org/10.1080/16549716.2019.1585709

Familiar, I., Muniina, P. N., Dolan, C., Ogwal, M., Serwadda, D., Kiyingi, H., Bahinduka, C. S., Sande, E., & Hladik, W. (2021). Conflict-related violence and mental health among self settled Democratic Republic of Congo female refugees in Kampala, Uganda—A respondent driven sampling survey. *Conflict and Health, 15*(1), 42. https://doi.org/10.1186/s13031-021-00377-2

Fry, M. W., Skinner, A. C., & Wheeler, S. B. (2019). Understanding the relationship between male gender socialization and gender-based violence among refugees in sub-Saharan Africa. *Trauma, Violence & Abuse, 20*(5), 638–652. https://doi.org/10.1177/1524838017727009

Gebreyesus, T., Sultan, Z., Ghebrezghiabher, H. M., Singh, N., Tol, W. A., Winch, P. J., Davidovitch, N., & Surkan, P. J. (2019). Violence en route: Eritrean women asylum seekers experiences of sexual violence while migrating to Israel. *Health Care for Women International, 40*, 721–743. https://doi.org/10.1080/07399332.2019.1566336

Gebreyesus, T., Sultan, Z., Ghebrezghiabher, H. M., Tol, W. A., Winch, P. J., Davidovitch, N., & Surkan, P. J. (2018). Life on the margins: The experiences of sexual violence and exploitation among Eritrean asylum-seeking women in Israel. *BMC Women's Health, 18*(1), 135. https://doi.org/10.1186/s12905-018-0624-y

Gillespie, A., Seff, I., Caron, C., Maglietti, M. M., Erskine, D., Poulton, C., & Stark, L. (2022). The pandemic made us stop and think about who we are and what we want: Using intersectionality to understand migrant and refugee women's experiences of gender-based violence during COVID-19. *BMC Public Health, 22*(1), 1469. https://doi.org/10.1186/s12889-022-13866-7

Hossain, M., Pearson, R. J., McAlpine, A., Bacchus, L. J., Spangaro, J., Muthuri, S., Muuo, S., Franchi, G., Hess, T., Bangha, M., & Izugbara, I. (2020). Gender-based violence and its association with mental health among Somali women in a Kenyan refugee camp: A latent class analysis. *Journal of Epidemiology & Community Health, 75*(4), 327–334. https://doi.org/10.1136/jech-2020-214086

Inter-Agency Standing Committee. (2015). *Integrating gender-based violence interventions in humanitarian action: Reducing risk, promoting resilience, and aiding recovery*. https://interagencystandingcommittee.org/system/files/2021-03/IASC%20Guidelines%20for%20Integrating%20GenderBased%20Violence%20Interventions%20in%20Humanitarian%20Action%2C%202015pdf

Islam, M. M., Khan, M. N., & Rahman, M. M. (2022). Intimate partner abuse among Rohingya women and its relationship with their abilities to reject husbands' advances to unwanted sex. *Journal of Interpersonal Violence*. https://doi.org/10.1177/0886260521991299

Kim, E., Yun, M., & von Denkowski, C. (2022). Violence against North Korean refugee women: Doubly victimized by repatriation and premigration traumatic experiences. *Violence against Women, 28*(10), 2424–2447. https://doi.org/10.1177/10778012211032706

Kong, B. S., Gezimu, W., Demeke, A., & Duguma, A. (2023). Prevalence of rape and its predictors among female students attending elementary schools: In the case of Kule refugee camp, Gambella Southwest Ethiopia—A cross-sectional study. *International Journal of Reproductive Medicine, 2023*, 5559246. https://doi.org/10.1155/2023/5559246

Laughon, K., Montalvo-Liendo, N., Eaton, S., & Bassett, L. (2023). Health and safety concerns of female asylum seekers living in an informal migrant camp in Matamoros Mexico. *Journal of Advanced Nursing, 79*(5), 1830–1839. https://doi.org/10.1111/jan.15511

Lever, H., Ottenheimer, D., Teysir, J., Singer, E., & Atkinson, H. G. (2019). Depression, anxiety, post-traumatic stress disorder, and a history of pervasive gender-based violence among women asylum seekers who have undergone female genital mutilation/cutting: A retrospective case review. *Journal of Immigrant and Minority Health, 21*(3), 483–489. https://doi.org/10.1007/s10903-018-0782-x

Logie, C. H., Okumu, M., Mwima, S., Hakiza, R., Irungi, K. P., Kyambadde, P., Kironde, E., & Narasimhan, M. (2019). Social ecological factors associated with experiencing violence among urban refugee and displaced adolescent girls and young women in Kampala, Uganda: A cross-sectional study. *Conflict and Health, 13*, 60. https://doi.org/10.1186/s13031-019-0242-9

Mezzatesta Gava, M., Miquel, L., & Jarvis, G. E. (2022). Gender-based violence among refugee women referred to a Cultural Consultation Service in Montreal. *Transcultural Psychiatry, 59*(2), 202–213. https://doi.org/10.1177/13634615211043767

Muuo, S., Muthuri, S. K., Mutua, M. K., McAlpine, A., Bacchus, L. J., Ogego, H., Bangha, M., Hossain, M., & Izugbara, C. (2020). Barriers and facilitators to care-seeking among survivors of gender-based violence in the Dadaab refugee complex. *Sexual and Reproductive Health Matters, 28*(1), 1722404. https://doi.org/10.1080/26410397.2020.1722404

Nam, B., Kim, J. Y., Lee, Y., & Fedina, L. (2022b). Polyvictimization risk among North Korean refugee women in South Korea. *Journal of Interpersonal Violence*. https://doi.org/10.1177/08862605211005146

Nam, B., Lee, Y., Bright, C., & Negi, N. (2022a). Polyvictimization and psychological outcomes among North Korean refugee women. *Violence against Women, 28*(15–16), 3726–3741. https://doi.org/10.1177/10778012221088311

Odwe, G., Undie, C. C., & Obare, F. (2018). Attitudes toward help-seeking for sexual and gender-based violence in humanitarian settings: The case of Rwamwanja refugee settlement scheme in Uganda. *BMC International Health and Human Rights, 18*(1), 15. https://doi.org/10.1186/s12914-018-0154-6

Pérez-Vázquez, S., & Bonilla-Campos, A. (2023). Women refugee's perceptions, experiences and coping mechanisms in situations of sexual and gender-based violence (SGBV): A metasynthesis. *Trauma, Violence & Abuse*. https://doi.org/10.1177/15248380221126470

Phillimore, J., Pertek, S., Akyuz, S., Darkal, H., Hourani, J., McKnight, P., Ozcurumez, S., & Taal, S. (2022). We are forgotten: Forced migration, sexual and gender-based violence, and coronavirus disease-2019. *Violence against Women, 28*(9), 2204–2230. https://doi.org/10.1177/10778012211030943

Rodella Sapia, M. D., Wangmo, T., Dagron, S., & Elger, B. S. (2020). Understanding access to professional healthcare among asylum seekers facing gender-based violence: A qualitative study from a stakeholder perspective. *BMC International Health and Human Rights, 20*(1), 25. https://doi.org/10.1186/s12914-020-00244-w

Rometsch, C., Denkinger, J. K., Engelhardt, M., Windthorst, P., Graf, J., Gibbons, N., Pham, P., Zipfel, S., & Junne, F. (2020). Pain, somatic complaints, and subjective concepts of illness in traumatized female refugees who experienced violence by the "Islamic State" (IS). *Journal of Psychosomatic Research, 130*, 109931. https://doi.org/10.1016/j.jpsychores.2020.109931

Roupetz, S., Garbern, S., Michael, S., Bergquist, H., Glaesmer, H., & Bartels, S. A. (2020). Continuum of sexual and gender-based violence risks among Syrian refugee women and girls in Lebanon. *BMC Women's Health, 20*(1), 176. https://doi.org/10.1186/s12905-020-01009-2

Sharma, V., Amobi, A., Tewolde, S., Deyessa, N., & Scott, J. (2020a). Displacement-related factors influencing marital practices and associated intimate partner violence risk among Somali refugees in Dollo Ado, Ethiopia: A qualitative study. *Conflict and Health, 14*, 17. https://doi.org/10.1186/s13031-020-00267-z

Sharma, V., Papaefstathiou, S., Tewolde, S., Amobi, A., Deyessa, N., Relyea, B., & Scott, J. (2020b). Khat use and intimate partner violence in a refugee population: A qualitative study in Dolla Ado. *Ethiopia. BMC Public Health, 20*(1), 670. https://doi.org/10.1186/s12889-020-08837-9

Treves-Kagan, S., Peterman, A., Gottfredson, N. C., Villaveces, A., Moracco, K. E., & Maman, S. (2022). Love in the time of war: Identifying neighborhood-level predictors of intimate partner violence from a longitudinal study in refugee-hosting communities. *Journal of Interpersonal Violence*. https://doi.org/10.1177/0886260520986267

Um, M. Y., Kim, H. J., & Palinkas, L. A. (2018). Correlates of domestic violence victimization among North Korean refugee women in South Korea. *Journal of Interpersonal Violence, 33*(13), 2037–2058. https://doi.org/10.1177/0886260515622297

Um, M. Y., Lee, J. O., Kim, H. J., Rice, E., & Palinkas, L. A. (2021). Testing the pathway from premigration sexual violence to suicide-related risk among North Korean refugee women living in South Korea: Do social networks matter? *Social Psychiatry and Psychiatric Epidemiology, 56*(3), 485–495. https://doi.org/10.1007/s00127-020-01977-8

United Nations High Commissioner for Refugees. (2020). *UNHCR policy on the prevention of, risk mitigation, and response to gender-based violence*. https://www.unhcr.org/media/unhcr-policy-prevention-risk-mitigation-and-response-gender-based-violence-2020-pdf

United Nations High Commissioner for Refugees. (2023b, June 14). *Refugee data finder*. https://www.unhcr.org/refugee-statistics/

United Nations High Commissioner for Refugees. (2023a). *Global trends: Forced displacement in 2022*. https://www.unhcr.org/global-trends-report-2022

Wachter, K., Horn, R., Friis, E., Falb, K., Ward, L., Apio, C., Wanjiku, S., & Puffer, E. (2018). Drivers of intimate partner violence against women in three refugee camps. *Violence against Women, 24*(3), 286–306. https://doi.org/10.1177/1077801216689163

Wikholm, K., Mishori, R., Ottenheimer, D., Korostyshevskiy, V., Reingold, R., Wikholm, C., & Hampton, K. (2020). Female genital mutilation/cutting as grounds for asylum requests in the US: An analysis of more than 100 cases. *Journal of Immigrant and Minority Health, 22*(4), 675–681. https://doi.org/10.1007/s10903-020-00994-8

Wringe, A., Yankah, E., Parks, T., Mohamed, O., Saleh, M., Speed, O., Hémono, R., Relyea, B., Ibrahim, M., Sandhu, J. S., & Scott, J. (2019). Altered social trajectories and risks of violence among young Syrian women seeking refuge in Turkey: A qualitative study. *BMC Women's Health, 19*(1), 9. https://doi.org/10.1186/s12905-019-0710-9

Into the Manosphere

8

Surea Gainey

Abstract

This section delves into the Red Pill community, also known as the "Manosphere," which originated as an online network designed to support young people facing challenges with building meaningful relationships. Over time, this online community has developed into a rigid system of social hierarchies led by charismatic leaders and self-proclaimed dating experts. Despite facing bans for its controversial viewpoints, the Manosphere has maintained a strong presence across social media platforms thanks to its viral content and adaptable marketing strategies. This online community conceals misogyny and alt-right conservatism as male-empowerment and preservationism; claiming that women's empowerment is directly responsible for male disenfranchisement and loneliness in today's world. These spaces exploit the vulnerabilities of men in distress, promoting archaic notions of masculinity as a solution to social and economic challenges. This chapter will delve into the fundamental beliefs of the Manosphere, provide a brief history of the reactionary movement, and propose interventions for individuals affected by feelings of isolation and excessive internet use.

Keywords

Manosphere • Toxic masculinity • Gender dynamics • Patriarchy • Misogyny • Sexism • Social hierarchies • Online communities • Gender dynamics • Gender inequality • Intersectionality • Power structures • Incel subculture • Social media • Alt-right radicalism • Red-pill ideology

S. Gainey (✉)
University of South Florida, Tampa, FL, USA
e-mail: sureagainey@gmail.com

S. Spowart (ed.), *Global Happiness and Humanitarian Assistance*, Integrated Science 29, https://doi.org/10.1007/978-3-031-71789-5_8

In recent years, a plague of pandemic proportions has been sweeping up unsuspecting victims across the globe. At a time when people have more opportunities to connect than ever before, many are finding it exceedingly difficult to do so, often with grave consequences. According to the U.S. Surgeon General, the loneliness epidemic requires a public health intervention similar to that of tobacco, obesity, and substance abuse (Office of the Assistant Secretary for Health, 2023). A silent killer, loneliness affects the young and the old, the affluent and the indigent indiscriminately. But before the lockdowns of the COVID-19 pandemic, most could not have predicted the degree to which loneliness would saturate our daily lives. In 2020, as March gave way to April and May, the compounding effects of our isolation became more prominent in our minds and bodies. Experts have shown that prolonged social isolation poses a significant risk for the development of mental health conditions like depression and anxiety (Office of the Surgeon General, 2023). Lack of social connection has been associated with the development of chronic diseases like heart disease, stroke, dementia, and even premature death (Office of the Surgeon General, 2023). The rise in the number of lonely, isolated individuals is a public health crisis befitting the second decade of the new millennium. Unfortunately for us, twenty years into the digital age have done little to prepare us for this new reality.

With the rise of government enforced lockdowns and closed schools, the youth have been turning increasingly to social media, virtual reality, and artificial intelligence technologies in search of a connection. In the early days of strict stay-at-home orders, many netizens took to the internet to educate themselves on the looming threats with varied results. According to Statista, the pandemic saw a rapid shift in consumption from traditional media like television to digital web and mobile platforms (Guttman, 2024). The trends have been on an incline ever since. In 2021, the average U.S. adult spent 485 min (over 8 h) engaging with digital content (Guttman, 2024). This number has continued to rise with current figures in 2024 averaging 508 min (almost 8.5 h) (Guttmann, 2024). With its infinite search results, the internet has been both a useful tool and an impractical adversary in the war against disinformation.

As Generation Z gives way to Generation Alpha, we are now bearing witness to two generations whose lives have been defined chiefly by their access to the internet. There is an internet culture, internet slang, and an absurdist sense of humor that could only be understood through the lens of decades of habitual internet use. Millions of people share their most private and personal stories with strangers online and receive an outpouring of sympathy in return. When they struggle to achieve the same connection offline, this reinforces where the sense of community really lies. Research has only just begun to examine how immersion in this technology from birth can affect our social development. For example, having extended hours of screen time has been linked to developmental delays, decreased communicative abilities and problem-solving skills in children as young as toddlers (Takahashi, et al., 2023). Not surprisingly, other researchers have found that reduced screen time and viewing content with a parent (particularly educational content) is associated with positive language learning outcomes in children (Madigan, et al. 2020). This is something to keep in mind when you consider that the United States lags behind other countries in media literacy despite ranking higher in terms of technology-based civic engagement (Media Literacy Now, 2021).

There are notable differences in how men and women use the internet as well. In the study How Women and Men Use the Internet, the Pew Research Center describes how unmarried men in particular report spending more hours online than unmarried women. The report also showed that men are more likely than women to use the internet as a vehicle for advice on personal matters such as politics, finances, and their careers (Pew Research Center, 2020). Men are significantly more likely than women to maintain their computers, engage in the latest trends across internet domains, and test new applications and features (Pew Research Center, 2020). Women were shown to be more apprehensive towards this technology due to its use in criminal activity and susceptibility to online harassment (Pew Research Center, 2020).

One corner of the web that has taken this demographic of young single men by storm is the male blogosphere known as the Manosphere. The Manosphere, a diverse network of content forums dedicated to discussing masculinity, men's issues, and the male lifestyle. With roots dating back to the dawn of the internet age, this vast media network has devolved into a battlefield of competing gender ideologies, controversial influencers, and fanatical fans. Unlike other online communities with limited social appeal, the Manosphere has established itself as a phenomenon offline by bringing its most controversial members to the forefront of an evolving discussion on men's rights. While it has remained relatively obscure enough to grant key figures the occasional platform on early morning breakfast shows, some of their most high-profile members have attracted international scrutiny for their divisiveness and adjacent criminal activity. With its liberal use of misogynistic dog-whistles and deep ties to white nationalist circles, the Manosphere has inspired a new generation of terrorists with a victim toll currently spanning across several countries in North America and Europe.

The internet's strength is that it is bursting with opportunities for social engagement. But with the rise of social media, the availability of harmful misinformation could spell disaster for lonely young men and boys who are particularly susceptible to such radicalization. Without discernment, the lack of safeguards for this technology could result in an individual adopting maladaptive coping strategies that put themselves and society at risk. We must learn to recognize the risks that misogynistic online communities pose to prevent them from erupting into greater health issues and social disharmony. In this section, we will outline the basic tenants of the Manosphere, examine its deadly impact, and prescribe possible remedies for men suffering from the crippling effects of loneliness and internet addiction.

1 Into the Manosphere

The Manosphere is a diverse genre of online content, blogs, and forums dedicated to discussing the dating, romantic, and sociocultural complexities of being a man. In her article for the Washington Post, Caitlin Dewey summarized the philosophies of the Manosphere in twofold: (1) The belief that 100 years of feminism has upset the natural order by making women equal to men. (2) Men can best save society by returning to traditional gender roles which reinforce the role of women as secondary helpmates. Described Eva Bujalka and Ben Rich for The Conversation, "[the Manosphere] contrasts the growing challenges faced by men with the increasing social, economic and political success experienced by women." This zero-sum game positions women's empowerment as the primary cause of male disempowerment, as evidenced by arcane, pseudoscientific theories of biology, psychology, and socioeconomics (Bujalka & Rich, 2023). For those men who fear the loss of their identity under a label-free society, the fear of their slow fade into irrelevancy is easily exploited by Manosphere opportunists who offer them a scapegoat for their struggles.

The Manosphere's impact on the culture can be felt in several ways, most noticeably in the rise of stochastic and misogynistic terrorist attacks over the last 10 years. In 2014, Manosphere zealot Elliot Rodger gained national attention when he executed a vengeful killing spree in Isla Vista, California. In his 141-page manifesto, the self-proclaimed "incel" (involuntarily celibate) pointed to the social and romantic rejection he felt at the hands of women as the catalyst for this "Day of Retribution". As someone who felt excluded from romance, Elliot's twisted solution required eradicating the objects of his affection who he felt had robbed him of the joys of human connection. Reminiscing on his numerous failed attempts at flirting, Elliot describes his motivation in his own words, "I had nothing left to live for but revenge. Women must be punished for their crimes of rejecting such a magnificent gentleman as myself." But Elliot also stressed the need to punish romantically successful men too. "All of those popular boys must be punished for enjoying heavenly lives and having sex with all the girls while I had to suffer in lonely virginity…. If I can't have it, I will destroy it." Elliot would later carry out his ultimate fantasy by killing 6 people, injuring 14 and fatally shooting himself. Alarmingly though, within the Manosphere chatrooms and message boards he had frequented, some began to canonize the terrorist as a saint, a hero, and the one true "Supreme Gentleman" (Witt, 2020).

Elliot Rodger is merely one example of how someone can become radicalized through a combination of social isolation and toxic online habits. But this instance of a nondescript young man committing a vicious attack before being venerated as a saint by his peers is only a small fraction of the devotees that can be found across the Manosphere.

2 Creating the Matrix

While I will be referring to the Manosphere as a single entity, it is more accurately imagined as a diverse web of communities each possessing a distinct perspective on men's roles in society. Nonetheless, certain beliefs can be found across all spheres.

Manosphere individuals identify each other based on a series of cultural references, the most famous coming from the 1999 film The Matrix. The Manosphere adopted the film's central metaphor of a disillusioned young man trapped inside a false reality as a symbol of the futility of the human experience. At a crossroads in his destiny, the main character, Neo, faces two life paths represented through the device of two pills. The first pill, blue, would allow Neo to avoid discovering the ugly truth about the world and ignore this reality while slipping seamlessly back into his daily life. The second pill, red, would enable him to view the world for what it truly is and fight on his terms. Within the Manosphere, the act of "taking the red pill" represents discovering the truth about heterosexual relationships. The "Red Pill" community's version of the truth is that romantic relationships are inherently transactional and that women have historically and continue to use sex and reproduction as a device to control men's lives. They cite history as proof of this fact. In historically patriarchal societies, sex and children were some of the intended outcomes of a marriage between a man and a woman. Under this system, men could demonstrate their success through their social and economic achievements, while women granted them the distinction of marriage and a legacy through children. The Manosphere argues that feminism has stripped marriage of the traditional benefits that come with being the primary breadwinner through the promises of gender equality. Blurring the lines between masculine and feminine roles and responsibilities. This shift in social dynamics is the supposed cause for the rise in depression, loneliness, and sexlessness in young men today.

With the rise of dating apps, women now possess as much (if not more) of the power of selection as men once did. A study showed that heterosexual men encompass more than 60% of the users on dating apps with men initiating the first contact at three times the rate of women (Matos, 2023). Manosphere adherents would argue that because we are living in a more equal and sexually permissive culture, women's priorities have shifted away from being dutiful wives and mothers to promiscuous pleasure seekers. Sex in the Manosphere is a stand in for control in a relationship. For a man to escape the Matrix, he must use his masculinity and "red pill awareness" to trick a woman into having sex on his terms with the least amount of commitment possible. Women under this system lose a piece of their value with every new sexual partner while the opposite is true for men. Special recognition is given to men who have frequent sex with multiple women. As such, a large swath of Manosphere content is dedicated to pick-up and seduction tactics for the young and inexperienced to amass praise and build on their masculinity.

Those who do not subscribe to this way of thinking are known to be Blue-pilled, more commonly known as beta males. In this model of subordinate masculinity, men who choose not to focus on competition and sexual exploits are written off as wimpish (Jewkes, et al., 2015). Compared to their red-pill counterparts, blue-pillers view recent advancements in women's reproductive, educational, and financial equality as a net benefit for society. Those opposing this view purport that because these opportunities also grant women the ability to outperform men in some areas, then gender inequality either cannot exist under feminism or the pendulum has swung too far in the opposite direction resulting in male disenfranchisement.

Some factions of the Manosphere believe civil liberties like no-fault divorce and spousal/child support are incentives for divorce that undermine male authority in the home. The fear of losing control of your family, assets, and freedom has driven some of these groups to a more drastic conclusion. MGTOW (Men Going Their Own Way) is one such online faction that advocates for a separatist movement of the genders. This could include refusing to date, befriend, or interact with women whenever possible. Some members of MGTOW limit female interaction to only direct family members while others may choose to stop interacting with women completely. While individuals subscribing to MGTOW often profess the benefits of decentering the female gaze, in reality, their persistent infatuation with women has led to them being associated with multiple online harassment campaigns (Galla, 2022).

The Manosphere also has strong ties to the Men's Rights Movement. While varied in their course of action, at the most basic level, men's rights activists (MRAs) fight for the legal rights of men and the pursuit of legal equality between the sexes. This could include bringing attention to instances of sex-based discrimination, domestic abuse, and legal inequalities faced by men in the court system. However, to make their case for marginalization, many MRAs embellish their claims of persecution by citing popular culture and celebrity' examples while insisting the same mistreatment is happening to all men an institutional level. According to the Southern Poverty Law Center (SPLC), men's rights groups often distort statistics to support their claims of female privilege and scapegoat women for the moral decay of society. Some choose to highlight male discrimination in STEM fields by weaponizing litigation against women-owned and women-oriented business models (Levintova, 2016). Others go even further and seek to intimidate victims of sexual assault by harassing women online, posting their pictures, and providing legal guidance for accused rapists (Scheinman, 2017). With the nebulous objective of fighting against male inequality, issues with far-reaching consequences like the male suicide rate and the underdiagnosis of mental health problems often come second to their primary goal of combatting feminism.

Most concerning is the Manosphere's hypothetical third option between the red and blue pill, which encompasses Incels and those who subscribe to the "Black Pill". This is the faction that inspired the likes of Elliot Rodger and others to commit unspeakable acts of violence. Playing on the analogy from The Matrix, the Involuntary Celibacy (Incel) community represents the fatalistic view of the world, but it did not start that way. According to the woman who coined the term in a 1990s message board, the Incel community was originally intended to be an inclusive safe space for men and women alike who struggled with loneliness, social anxiety, and a lack of social connections (Kassam, 2018). It has since devolved into an extremist sect of the Manosphere that the Southern Poverty Law Center has classified as a male supremacist hate group.

Incels and black-pillers adhere to a strict looks-based hierarchy which they believe determines not only their ability to maintain relationships but friendships as well. Black pill content contains elements of Social Darwinism, scientific racism, and biological determinism. Incels like Rodgers used these theories on genetic fitness to relegate women to the role of natural selectors and incels as genetic failures. Where the red pillers seek to reassert dominance over women through traditional gender roles and economic means of persuasion (Van Valkenburgh, 2018), black-pillers view their loneliness as a permanent condition, adopting the common phrase "it's over" as an acceptance that they were stamped from birth as romantic rejects (Preston et al., 2021).

One fatal day in April 2018, 19-year-old Alek Minassian chose to execute his "final mission", a mission which he believed would continue his idol's legacy and inspire others like him to rise up in solidarity. Embittered by his lack of sexual experience and the success of men he considered "brutes", Minassian grew to believe that only an act of terrorism would end the suffering of men like himself, a phenomenon known as a "beta uprising" or "Incel Rebellion". In a Facebook post written by Minassian hours before the attack, he made the following statements: "The Incel Rebellion has already begun! We will overthrow all the Chads and Stacys! All hail the Supreme Gentleman Elliot Rodger!" (Coletta, 2019). Soon after making this post, Minassian deliberately drove his vehicle onto a crowded Toronto sidewalk and accelerated, killing 10 people and injuring 16 (Coletta, 2019). In a later interview with a detective, Minassian would say that he felt other Incels were "too cowardly" to act on their anger and that he was satisfied he had "accomplished [his] mission" (Coletta, 2019). Like his friend Elliot (whom Alek had close contact with leading up to the 2014 attack in Isla Vista, California) Minassian had become radicalized from a combination of social isolation and toxic online computer habits.

Contrary to these narratives found within the Manosphere, the loneliness epidemic has not been linked to rampant misandry brought on by feminism. In reality, with the growing acceptance of women's social equality, some men have found it difficult to adapt to a world where opportunities for connection are rare, the dating standards of women are high, and gender is now a theoretical construct. But in this highly ambiguous world, what it means to be a "real" man is an increasingly subjective experience which we can see reflected in the burgeoning array of gender representation in traditional and unconventional media alike.

3 Masculinity: A Biological Reality or a Set of Rules?

Webster's Dictionary defines masculinity as the qualities associated with men and boys; But since these attributes vary widely across time and space, how much of that is socially constructed versus biologically determined has been the source of some debate. Using the Social Identity Theory, masculinity can be understood as both a self-imposed identity and an simplification of human behavior (Islam, 2014). In R.W. Connell's essay The Social Organization of Masculinity, she argues that gender is a social construct based on functionality, anatomy, and the responsibilities of everyday life. For that reason, Connell theorized that masculinity is not a biological trait, but a spectrum of different identities dependent on time, location, and the individual environment. Connell later used these theories to describe a hierarchy of masculinity based on proximity to the norm.

Hegemonic Masculinity describes the dominant form of masculinity recognized by a society. In the West, this may describe a man who embodies themes of Grecian stoicism, traditional athleticism, sexual attractiveness, and wealth. Within the Manosphere, the terms "alpha male" and "Chad" are used to describe men who are physically attractive, sexually desirable, and high in social currency (Brooks et al., 2022). This version of masculinity is so ubiquitious that being a traditional protector and provider in this system is seen as an embrace of traditional Western values. In R.W. Connell's framework, the Manosphere's definition of masculinity is just one of potentially hundreds present in throughout human history. Many Incels and black-pillers suffer from depression due to a perceived lack of hegemonic masculinity, innocently believing that there is only one way for men to be given the dominance of this archetype in the media. Throughout his manifesto, Elliot Rodger detailed the numerous ways in which he sought to gain favor from his peers; This included buying expensive clothes, driving luxury cars, and attempting to flirt and socialize with girls at parties. It was his failure to meet this version of manhood that made Rodger susceptible to the deafening rhetoric of the Manosphere, which classifies romantic relationships as the ultimate form of social capital. In a society that upholds traditional hegemonic norms, a woman's primary role is to support the men in her life and reaffirm their value through acts of submission. In this way, female subjugation aids in the perpetuation of the male identity. To emancipate a woman would be in direct defiance of the roles outlined for women throughout modern history. Under the current conditions of the twentieth century, the hegemonic principle is no longer valid.

4 A Bitter Alternative

In the absence of external opinions, many men of the Manosphere become entangled in what is known as the Alt-Right radicalization pipeline. A genre of content designed to desensitize people to racism, sexism, populism, homophobia, and anti-progressive values. Incels in particular are susceptible to social theories on race, as evidenced by their usage of racialized identity markers like "rice-cel" and "curry-cel" to describe East Asian and South Asian incels specifically (Ware, 2021). Wrote Aja Romano for her Vox news article titled How the alt-right's sexism lures men into white supremacy, "for many of its members, the gateway drug that led them to join the alt-right in the first place wasn't racist rhetoric but rather sexism: extreme misogyny evolving from male bonding gone haywire." In his book

Angry White Men: American Masculinity at the End of an Era, Michael Kimmell describes how members of previously dominant groups (specifically straight white males) have found themselves increasingly disempowered by the end of unquestioned, unchallenged male authority. Their response to the growing social equality of minorities has been to regress to previous models of social inequality where racial and gender hierarchies were strictly enforced.

The sense of aggrieved entitlement, which Kimmel defines as the fear of losing privileges you believe you are entitled to, is pervasive throughout Red Pill and Black Pill spaces. It is also a useful tool for far-right reactionaries looking for ways to mobilize angry populations for their cause. In his book, Devil's Bargain, Joshua Green describes how Donald Trump's chief strategist, Steve Bannon, sought to engage "rootless white males" with deep roots in online gaming communities to support his nationalist agenda during the 2016 presidential election (Barro and Friedman, 2017). By targeting "motivated gamers" and "message-board denizens", Bannon was able to align himself with the most disciplined, fanatical, and insular online communities (Green, 2018). By appealing to the anger of this population, Bannon successfully mobilized an army of internet trolls and activists to drive online engagement around presidential hopeful Donald Trump in 2016 (Green, 2018). Since 2016, this formula has been used to spawn a generation of Manosphere-adjacent influencers, like vaccine conspiracist Alex Jones and political commentator Ben Shapiro, who both hold strong anti-feminist views. For younger audiences, media personalities like Sneako (real name Nicolas "Nico" Kenn De Balinthazy) and Andrew Tate have gained followings of millions while openly condoning violence against women (Das, 2022), minorities, and the LBGTQ + (Wiggins, 2023). When these views earn them a ban from larger platforms like YouTube, Twitch, and TikTok, their devoted armies of followers follow them to far-right platforms like Rumble which are built around insular communities peddling fake products and conspiracy theories (Farah, 2023).

Across the Manosphere, there is a consistent wave of support given to those who challenge women's bodily autonomy offline as well. When Alabama instituted abortion penalties that were harsher on the women seeking treatment than the men accused of assault, male supremacist groups applauded the move (SPLC, 2023). In California, one self-proclaimed incel gathered a significant following on Youtube by filming himself assaulting women and uploading the evidence online (Haas, 2022). He was later apprehended while hiding in his self-titled "rape van" after his videos went viral for harassment (Haas, 2022).

This sentimentality for a bygone era of boys-will-be-boys is not a response unique to modern social movements. In his book God's Politics: Why the Right Gets It Wrong and the Left Doesn't Get It, Jim Wallis describes the types of conditions that breed fundamentalist movements. Said Wallis, "Fundamentalism is essentially a revolt against modernity. It is a reaction based on profound fear and defensiveness against 'losing the faith.'" (Wallace, 66). With this idea in mind, it's not difficult to imagine how a rapidly progressing society has the potential to incur backlash as a result of the old faith being lost. But the rule of life does not have to be a zero-sum game.

From a social perspective, spaces like the Manosphere can provide invaluable opportunities for community and fellowship. The benefit of having a space where like-minded people can form an identity based on a shared narrative isn't inherently harmful. It has the potential to be an invaluable resource for young men in search of a solution for their social woes. However, for that to happen, we must address the root cause of the bitterness that's currently sending misguided men spiraling down a path of self-destruction.

5 Unplugging from the Matrix

At first glance, the reactionary views that make up the Manosphere could be written off solely as a collection of embittered social pariahs lashing out after a century of social progressivism. However, upon a closer look, this phenomenon and others like it has deep roots in the way we use technology to connect with the world and each other. The internet has democratized access to information, eliminated the geographical barriers that divide us, and revolutionized the way we commiserate on a global scale. At the same time, it has contributed to the rapid spread of disinformation and given rise to countless informational silos and (echo chambers) where individuals are exposed to content that reinforces their preexisting beliefs. Ironically, the anonymity and accessibility of the internet have contributed to the further polarization of our society and discouraged critical thinking among its chronic users.

The epidemic of lonely, isolated young men has become an ever-present threat to the greater health and well-being of our society. After examining the motivations of the Manosphere, there are three main reasons why I believe young men are turning to toxic ideologies instead of learning to cope constructively:

1. **We are spending an increasing amount of time alone and online**

Young men spend more time online using the internet than their female counterparts (Pew Research Center, 2020). Chronic loneliness has proven adverse health effects (Office of the Surgeon General, 2023) which can leave young men susceptible to the self-limiting beliefs of the Manosphere. It is essential to recognize the signs of chronic internet abuse to intervene at the first signs of dependency.

2. **The life scripts we have been raised with are becoming increasingly outdated**

Striving for a bygone era where limits on self expression were viewed as the foundation of society is, at best, a misguided use of nostalgia and at worst an exercise in futility that can exacerbate symptoms of depression. With the rising cost of living, inflation, and wage stagnation, the traditional male role of being the sole protector and provider has become increasingly elusive. Therefore, it is befitting that our concepts of masculinity adjust with the times to reflect the current changes in gender dynamics both within and outside the home.

3. **The Manosphere taps into an under utilized male perspective**

Traditional media has failed to charitably represent the unique social, psychological, and economic implications surrounding men's mental health and emotional well-being in a feminist world. Neglecting this perspective can have devastating effects on men's self-determination which the Manosphere capitalizes on by promoting their regressive outlook. Preventing frustrated young men and boys from turning to toxic ideologies requires an intersectional lens that critically examines the dynamic relationships between men, women, gender, income, and socio-cultural factors in a society.

The following solutions have the potential to support men in meeting their social, mental, and emotional goals:

1. **Treat the symptoms of technology dependency and economic stagnation without stigma or judgment**

This may involve investing in mental health resources and bringing awareness to the growing number of health issues that accompany habitual computer use. Encourage intimate and platonic friendships between boys at an early age and emphasize the importance of maintaining these relationships throughout the lifespan. The western hegemonic lifestyle tends to overstate the value of financial security as a prerequisite for dating and social lives. However, high rates of unemployment and cost of living have substantially limited men's abilities to perform patriarchy and socialize offline. More should be done by therapists and sociological professionals to explore these fears and meet the demands for positive online experiences instead of ignoring this new reality or falling back onto old scripts.

2. **Promote alternative forms of masculinity that do not involve women and dating**

While there are innumerable examples of men who do not fit the mold of a traditional "alpha male" and still have thriving personal lives, a cultural shift in acceptance towards alternative forms of gender expression must take place to cement this idea into the public psyche. The men of the Manosphere present a one-size-fits-all solution to success. But men who may not fit neatly into the traditional roles prescribed by the Manosphere may find a different lifestyle or philosophy more fulfilling. By embracing other forms of masculinity, ones that take into consideration gender as a social construct, we can grow to recognize and appreciate the natural gradient of masculinities present throughout human society.

3. **Provide personalized, concrete advice instead of general platitudes that do nothing to help promote social awareness**

Much of the dating and relationship advice we give to lonely, socially awkward men is too general to be of value in our rapidly changing world. For example, telling someone with social anxiety and depression to just "be themselves" around women is not going to be helpful in their journey of self-improvement. It is important to remember that what we lack in constructive criticism, the Manosphere makes up for in its sophisticated pick-up artistry and game-by-game playbooks for social interactions. Raising awareness around how depression manifests in men and deprogramming the harmful side effects of toxic masculinity through tailored guidance, increased clarity, and emotional support can drastically improve one's self-esteem and perspective.

6 Life after the Matrix

The United States has undergone major cultural changes over the past 100 years. Two decades into the digital age have given us a glimpse of what can happen if we allow technology to replace our desire for social interaction. In the age of social distancing, the internet has irreparably changed the way we approach the search for human connection. This quarantine-style approach has led to the rise of insular communities like Manosphere where men are plied with pseudoscientific platitudes about human nature in order to keep them desperate and pliable to gurus and grifters. On the surface, the Manosphere's messages of self-determination in the face of institutional neglect can seem empowering, but the underlying tone of power and control over lesser groups quickly diminishes any claims of disenfranchisement at the hands of the system. Nonetheless, because of the quasi-empowering nature of these groups, we must approach criticizing the Manosphere with extreme caution. While the Manosphere can perpetuate the harmful ideologies of toxic masculinity, it can also offer a sense of visibility and hope that is reflected in its popular influencers, millions of followers, and billions of views.

To circumvent the epidemic of loneliness we must reinforce the communicative ties that have led to this breakdown between the sexes, society, and our perception of our place within these constructs. This new chapter of the information age will incorporate the inclusive messaging of the past 20 years and build towards a new future where everyone, regardless of gender, feels empowered and informed to lead happier, healthier lives.

References

Barro, J., & Friedman, N. (2017). Here's how steve bannon used angry white gamers to build himself up to trump's chief strategist. *Business Insider*, www.businessinsider.com/steve-bannon-white-gamers-seinfeld-joshua-green-donald-trump-devils-bargain-sarah-palin-world-warcraft-gamergate-2017-7

Brooks, R. C., et al. (2022). Incel activity on social media linked to local mating ecology. *Psychological Science, 33*(2), 249–258. https://doi.org/10.1177/09567976211036065

Bujalka, E., Rich, B. (2023). Senior lecturer in history and international relations, The draw of the 'manosphere': Understanding Andrew Tate's appeal to lost men. *The Conversation*, theconversation.com/the-draw-of-the-manosphere-understanding-andrew-tates-appeal-to-lost-men-199179

Coletta, A. (2019). Toronto van attack: Minassian told police his 'mission' was ... *The Washington Post*, www.washingtonpost.com/world/the_americas/man-accused-of-killing-10-in-toronto-van-attack-told-police-his-mission-was-accomplished/2019/09/27/d5152a44-e161-11e9-be7f-4cc85017c36f_story.html

Connell, R. W. (2016). The social organization of masculinity. *Feminist Theory Reader*, 5th ed.

Das, S. (2022, 6 Aug) Inside the violent, Misogynistic world of Tiktok's new Star, Andrew Tate. *The Guardian*, Guardian News and Media, www.theguardian.com/technology/2022/aug/06/andrew-tate-violent-misogynistic-world-of-tiktok-new-star

Dewey, C. (2014) Inside the 'Manosphere' that inspired Santa Barbara shooter ... *Washington Post*, www.washingtonpost.com/news/the-intersect/wp/2014/05/27/inside-the-manosphere-that-inspired-santa-barbara-shooter-elliot-rodger/

Farah, H. (2023, 20 Sept) What is rumble, the video-sharing platform 'immune to cancel culture'? *The Guardian*, Guardian News and Media, www.theguardian.com/technology/2023/sep/20/what-is-rumble-the-video-sharing-platform-immune-to-cancel-culture

Galla, S. (2022, 3 Feb) MGTOW: The ultimate guide to men going their own way movement. *MensGroup.Com*, Mensgroup.com/mgtow/#What_Exactly_is_MGTOW.

Green, J. (2018) *Devil's Bargain*. Random House USA

Guttmann, A. (2023, 29 Aug) Time spent with digital media in the U.S. 2024. *Statista*, www.statista.com/statistics/262340/daily-time-spent-with-digital-media-according-to-us-consumsers/

Haas, G. (2022, 12 Oct) Incel' hate crime suspect faces charges in California connected to Youtube videos. *KLAS*, KLAS, www.8newsnow.com/news/local-news/incel-hate-crime-suspect-faces-charges-in-california-connected-to-youtube-videos/

Islam, G. (2014). Social identity theory. *Encyclopedia of Critical Psychology*. https://doi.org/10.1007/978-1-4614-5583-7_289

Jewkes, R., et al. (2015). Hegemonic masculinity: Combining theory and practice in gender interventions. *Culture Health Sexuality, 17*(sup2), 112–127. https://doi.org/10.1080/13691058.2015.1085094

Kassam, A. (2018, 26 Apr) Woman behind 'Incel' says angry men hijacked her word as a weapon of war. *The Guardian*, Guardian News and Media, www.theguardian.com/world/2018/apr/25/woman-who-invented-incel-movement-interview-toronto-attack

Kimmel, M. (2019). *Angry White Men: American Masculinity at the End of an Era*. Bold Type Books.

Levintova, H. (2016, 15 Jan) These men's rights activists are suing women's groups for meeting without men. *Mother Jones*, www.motherjones.com/politics/2016/01/men-rights-unruh-act-women-discrimination/

Madigan, S., et al. (2020). Associations between screen use and Child language skills. *JAMA Pediatrics, 174*(7), 665. https://doi.org/10.1001/jamapediatrics.2020.0327

Male Supremacy. (n.d.) *Southern Poverty Law Center*, www.splcenter.org/fighting-hate/extremist-files/ideology/male-supremacy

Marsh, K. (n.d.). How Lonely Single Men Can Redefine Love. *Psychology Today*, Sussex Publishers, www.psychologytoday.com/us/blog/the-state-of-our-unions/202212/how-lonely-single-men-can-redefine-love

Matos, G. (2023) The harsh reality men face on dating apps. *Psychology Today*, Sussex Publishers, www.psychologytoday.com/us/blog/the-state-of-our-unions/202305/the-harsh-reality-men-face-on-dating-apps

Office of the Surgeon General (OSG). (2023). Our Epidemic of Loneliness and Isolation: The U.S. Surgeon General's Advisory on the Healing Effects of Social Connection and Community [Internet]. Washington (DC): US Department of Health and Human Services, PMID: 37792968

Office of the Assistant Secretary for Health (OASH). (2023, 3 May) New Surgeon General Advisory Raises Alarm about the Devastating Impact of the Epidemic of Loneliness and Isolation in the United States. *HHS.Gov*, www.hhs.gov/about/news/2023/05/03/new-surgeon-general-advisory-raises-alarm-about-devastating-impact-epidemic-loneliness-isolation-united-states.html#:~:text=Vivek%20Murthy%20released%20a%20new,experiencing%20measurable%20levels%20of%20loneliness

Pew Research Center. (2020, August 7). How Women and Men use the Internet | Pew Research Center: Internet, Science & Tech. https://www.pewresearch.org/internet/2005/12/28/how-women-and-men-use-the-internet/#:~:text=Issues%20about%20gender%20and%20the,more%20concerned%20about%20its%20risks

Preston, K., et al. (2021). The black pill: New technology and the male supremacy of involuntarily celibate men. *Men and Masculinities, 24*(5), 823–841. https://doi.org/10.1177/1097184x211017954

Romano, A. (2016, 14 Dec). How the alt-right's sexism lures men into white supremacy. *Vox*, www.vox.com/culture/2016/12/14/13576192/alt-right-sexism-recruitment

Scheinman, T. (2017). *Silencing Women: Inside the National Coalition for Men—Pacific Standard Magazine*, psmag.com/news/silencing-women-inside-national-coalition-men-rape-sexual-assault-harry-crouch-94284.

Takahashi, I., et al. (2023). Screen time at age 1 year and communication and problem-solving developmental delay at 2 and 4 years. *JAMA Pediatrics, 177*(10), 1039. https://doi.org/10.1001/jamapediatrics.2023.3057

US, (2021, 28 July). Media literacy rates still low: media literacy now. *Media Literacy Now Advocating for Media Literacy Education*, medialiteracynow.org/a-new-index-shows-that-he-us-scores-low-on-media-literacy-education/

Van Valkenburgh, S. P. (2018). Digesting the red pill: Masculinity and neoliberalism in the manosphere. *Men and Masculinities, 24*(1), 84–103. https://doi.org/10.1177/1097184x18816118

Wallis, J. (2009). *God's Politics: Why the Right Gets It Wrong and the Left Doesn't Get It.* HarperOne

Ware, J. (2021). *Beta Uprising is There an Incel Threat to Asia? On JSTOR*, www.jstor.org/stable/27016616

Wiggins, C. (2023, 19 Sept) Incel influencer Sneako's young fans yell 'all gays should die' in viral video. *Advocate.Com*, Advocate.com, www.advocate.com/media/disturbing-sneako-video-kids-transphobic

Witt, T. (2020). 'If I cannot have it, I will do everything I can to destroy it.' the canonization of Elliot Rodger: 'Incel' masculinities, secular sainthood, and justifications of ideological violence. *Social Identities, 26*(5), 675–689. https://doi.org/10.1080/13504630.2020.1787132

Surea Gainey holds a Master of Public Health degree from the University of South Florida, Tampa. A native of Fort Walton Beach, she is dedicated to dismantling institutional barriers and uncovering pre-existing biases with the goal of reshaping them to drive social change. Surea believes that compassion-driven solutions can enlighten minds and foster meaningful dialogue. In her first publication, she aims to challenge harmful and reductive narratives, shifting attention to the critical issues affecting our society.

Evaluation of Schizoid Personality Disorder: Background, Misconceptions, and the Interrelation with Violence

9

Casey Lewandowski

Abstract

Schizoid personality disorder is traditionally viewed as rare with a prevalence rate of less than 5%. Due to its classification as eccentric and odd, individuals with this disorder are incorrectly grouped into the realm of schizophrenia and other severe mental illnesses, which causes many misconceptions and further isolates these individuals from society. The disorder commonly presents as a lack of emotion and social isolation/detachment, yet, some erroneously believe that these individuals are "crazy" or "always violent" due to the fallacies surrounding this disorder. Hence, it becomes increasingly challenging for these individuals to engage with a culture that consistently portrays them degradingly. Therefore, this review aims to address these concerns and bring awareness to the true nature of schizoid personality disorder. There is an analysis of psychotherapy and pharmacotherapy as monotherapies and a reinforcing call for research regarding the combination of these therapies. Additionally, there is a discussion regarding comorbid disorders that, when properly managed, can aid in the reduction of schizoid symptoms. Furthermore, by calling on other researchers and practitioners to develop comprehensive treatment plans, more individuals will be able to get the help they need before their clinical manifestations harm themselves or others.

Keywords

DSM • Personality disorders • Schizoid • Therapies • Comorbidities • Violence • Literature review

C. Lewandowski (✉)
Department of Psychology, University of South Florida, Tampa, FL, USA
e-mail: clewandowski27@usf.edu

S. Spowart (ed.), *Global Happiness and Humanitarian Assistance*, Integrated Science 29, https://doi.org/10.1007/978-3-031-71789-5_9

1 Introduction

Known to researchers, psychologists, and clinical practitioners as a rare and complex condition, schizoid personality disorder (SzPD) lives up to its reputation. This disorder is best known for expressing little emotion and disengaging from social relationships. Individuals with this disorder prefer to be alone and are known to be indifferent to any form of recognition or disapproval. This disorder appears to be easily understood, though that is not the case. Research has shown that the majority of the people diagnosed with this disorder continually fit into the criteria outlined in the Diagnostic and Statistical Manual of Mental Disorders (DSM). However, there is also research based on first-hand accounts from people diagnosed with the disorder that highlight the differences in the typical patterns of SzPD and the misinterpretations that every diagnosed individual fits the criteria perfectly.

This paper aims to provide a background of SzPD while covering the presentation, prevalence, and etiology. The examination of current treatments and the need for more will take place. It is also important to note the additional emphasis on how SzPD impacts personality development. As foreshadowed earlier, SzPD is not one-size-fits-all. Unfortunately, due to the lack of research, if not poor research, SzPD is seen as precisely that. There is deficient accounting for the variation or deviation of typical symptoms and improper analysis of potential comorbidities, which can interfere with an accurate diagnosis.

Additionally, there are concerns about how mental disorders and violence in society are related. Therefore, this paper will also evaluate the relationship between SzPD and violence/violent tendencies. This discussion is paramount as there is confusion regarding the role of SzPD and its impact on violence. Societal comprehension of this disorder is very inadequate. Consequently, this contributes to the misconceptions regarding this disorder.

2 Background, Importance, and Literature Review

The worldwide prevalence rate of personality disorders (PDs) is estimated to be 7.8% (Winsper et al., 2020). According to the American Psychiatric Association (APA), the national prevalence rate for schizoid personality disorder in the United States ranges between 3.1 and 4.9% (APA, 2013). These numbers show that personality disorders, in general, are far from uncommon in the world itself and that SzPD is not irregular in the United States. With such an elevated prevalence, it is questionable how little the public understands this disorder. Understanding the presentation of SzPD is essential in resolving this issue. It can also provide further insight into the prevalence rates.

Individuals with SzPD exhibit a small range of emotional expressions, if at all (Căndel & Constantin, 2017). More often than not, they are emotionless in the eyes of others. Along these lines, there is a reduction in the pleasure derived from bodily, sensory, or interpersonal experiences (APA, 2013). This reduction in satisfaction means that, for example, sex will not please them as it would for others.

Although, it is a hallmark, or criterion, of the disorder to have little to no interest in sexual experiences with others (APA, 2013). However, it is not just intimate relationships but relationships in general that these individuals avoid. Social and close relationships apply to this avoidance, with the occasional exception of parents, full siblings, or children, also known as first-degree relatives (APA, 2013). While they have the potential to be around these relatives, they still lack the desire to form that intimate, close family bond. In these situations, they do not appear to take away enjoyment from these encounters. This avoidance and lack of pleasure are simply features of the disorder.

While they show persistent detachment from social relationships, they also prefer to spend time alone than with others (APA, 2013). Often described as loners, these individuals virtually always choose solitary activities and hobbies (APA, 2013). Since they lack close friends and do not want to interact with others, they turn to some form of computer or video game. Doing such an activity is due to their preference for abstract or mechanical tasks (APA, 2013). However, no matter how much they want to perform these activities, they may still not derive pleasure from them. In this case, the execution of the activities would merely pass the time. Nevertheless, these individuals remain isolated and have no involvement in the big things found in life (Stone, 1993).

Furthermore, these individuals are indifferent to recognition, approval, criticism, or disapproval. They are simply not bothered by how others view them (APA, 2013). To most, social cues can be very obvious. However, with SzPD, these individuals often appear oblivious to these cues and may not respond appropriately (APA, 2013). The typical abnormal expressions arise along the lines of self-absorption and superficiality. These individuals are dull in the eyes of many (Esterberg et al., 2010). According to the APA, they have a bland exterior with no visible emotional reactions and do not react physically with gestures (APA, 2013). People usually consider them to have a flat personality or be cold and emotionally unavailable. The APA also says these individuals seldom experience intense emotions (APA, 2013). Lastly, these individuals can reveal themselves in social settings but report a feeling of pain while doing so (APA, 2013). While they are brief, temporary moments, they are still highly uncommon.

In terms of their occupation, they experience impairment when interacting with others. Therefore, they often find jobs that they can perform alone. Additionally, when they experience stress, these individuals may also experience psychotic episodes (APA, 2013). It is even said to be an antecedent to delusional disorder or schizophrenia (APA, 2013). After all, there is the consideration that schizoid is a part of the schizophrenia spectrum disorders, with SzPD sitting on one end and schizophrenia being on the complete opposite side (Fariba et al., 2022).

Considering the etiology, SzPD makes its first appearance in childhood and adolescence. The hallmarks include isolation, poor relationships with peers, and poor performance in schooling (APA, 2013). How this disorder develops is still a mystery to researchers. The most prominent idea is the increase in the likelihood of inheriting the condition. The results of a study concluded that the genetic liability for SzPD is 26% (Kendler et al., 2006). A later investigation shows that this conclusion holds and that the schizophrenia spectrum disorders were all highly heritable (Kendler et al., 2007). Another substantial piece of etiology is that men receive more diagnoses for SzPD than women (APA, 2013; Klonsky et al., 2002). Other research supports these diagnostic differences through empirical analysis (Klonsky et al., 2002).

Additionally, there is massive debate on whether or not SzPD has an environmental factor. The DSM does not consider this factor to be a likely cause. However, a study shows that loneliness is a critical factor in the etiology of SzPD (Martens, 2010). Building on what the world knows about personality development, a connection appears between what the individual experienced in childhood and their presentation of the disorder. For example, if the primary caregiver was cold and detached during childhood, it is not unreasonable for the child to believe that relationships are unsatisfying. The child then follows this pattern and presents as cold and disconnected but with the added factor of displeasing and unsatisfying interactions with others. There is an enormous emphasis on how genetics impact personality development and the potential for disorders. However, the study of personality shows that the environment and other sociocultural facets influence how an individual's personality develops in their younger years. These influences can include parental and peer relationships, cultural impacts, the assessment and evaluation of others, and any physical aspects that impact them, such as abuse or other trauma. Regardless of the setting or behaviors, risk factors for the disorder are still present.

To most, individuals with this disorder simply prefer to keep to themselves and are satisfied with their lives. It appears nonchalant to many people, but that is a cause for concern. Empirical research on SzPD is severely restricted and thus significantly problematic. Unless the legal system or their families apply force, these individuals do not emerge in clinical environments for evaluation and diagnosis. The hallmarks of the disorder include not enjoying close relationships, appearing emotionally cold, showing detachment, and wanting isolation. Therefore, it is not surprising or unusual for these individuals to not show up voluntarily for clinical assessment; it represents their pattern of egosyntonic behavior. They see nothing wrong with their behavior, so they do not feel the need to modify anything. This evidence leads to the problem of not having a precise prevalence rate due to the underreporting of the disorder. From the reports that researchers have access to, a lower limit can be measured. However, having no explicit number only leads to the ambiguity of the true prevalence of SzPD.

The lack of data leads to many problems. First and foremost, it leads to a noticeable absence of research on SzPD. This deficiency of research could be the key to why there are no definitive answers as to the nature or cause of the disorder. With what little investigation is present, there is the additional problem of not controlling for other personality disorders or other comorbid conditions (e.g., antisocial personality disorder, substance use disorder, or depression). There is research saying that Asperger's syndrome is a potential risk factor for SzPD (Tantem, 1988). However, the point is that the analyses tie conditions together but do not fully control for the possibility of another co-occurring disorder being responsible for the expression of symptoms. These problems show poor and improper research but highlight the interference with an accurate diagnosis. If the knowledge of SzPD comes from research, but the studies themselves have errors, then the judgment of the clinical presentation has inherent room for fallacies.

The second problem arises consecutively from the first and accentuates how improper research leads to the enigma of SzPD treatments. Being under-researched compared to other PDs and mental health conditions is already problematic in general. Yet, this also means that treatments for SzPD are also under-researched. Not only is it demanding to find an effective treatment, but long-term follow-up research is a must to ensure adequate and sustainable treatment. Practitioners are aware of the imperfect sufficiency of a single intervention for their patients. Research on other conditions, such as depression, reveals that successful treatment of maladaptive behaviors may require a combination of therapy techniques or pharmacological interventions. For example, brexpiprazole is a monotherapy for schizophrenia but is an adjunctive pharmacotherapy treatment for major depressive disorder (Eaves & Rey, 2016). It prides itself on reducing depression symptoms by over fifty percent. While this is exceptional news, it shows what continued research can do. There was a call over a decade ago asking for more information on the efficacy of psychotherapy and pharmacotherapy combinations (Frank et al., 2005). Time has passed, but there are still calls asking for effective treatments and strategies concerning treatment combinations (Cuijpers et al., 2021). While these calls are towards the direction of depressive and anxiety disorders, there is still a need to evaluate new and effective treatments for PDs in general.

Currently, the treatment for personality disorders happens on a case-by-case basis with a highly tailored treatment plan. Everyone presents differently in a clinical setting, as their personality disorder has the potential to affect them differently than others. For SzPD, the primary treatment is psychotherapy. These therapies are cognitive-behavioral therapy (CBT), psychodynamic therapy, or dialectical behavioral therapy (DBT). CBT has the patient examine their thoughts, infer how they are troublesome, and redirect their beliefs with positive and productive thinking to promote better feelings and emotions. Psychodynamic therapy helps patients by helping to gain insight into their inner thoughts, actions, and desires. Diving deep into the unconscious shows the drivers of behaviors and brings awareness to who the person is. In doing so, the individual learns more about who they are and even discovers how to communicate better. DBT helps by having the patient realize their negative emotions and feelings, accept them, let them go, and provide the resources to help regulate future emotions and feelings. The emotional regulation gained allows the patient to move away from behaviors that could be harmful or self-destructive. As modern medicine and psychology hold, psychotherapy is the only treatment available.

Research shows little evidence regarding pharmacotherapy in SzPD (Koch et al., 2016). That is, medication cannot treat the disorder alone. However, prescription pharmaceuticals can treat comorbid conditions such as anxiety. Individuals with SzPD can have exposure to very little or too much stimulation and develop an anxiety disorder as a result (Esterberg et al., 2010). Additionally, due to their preferred lack of contact with others and the co-occurring symptom of emotional disengagement, their minds may wander into a fantasy world (Esterberg et al., 2010). This preoccupation with the imaginative world can lead to psychotic episodes, even if they are only brief (Esterberg et al., 2010). These episodes can lead to the potential prescription of anti-psychotics if they are frequent or worrisome. Along similar lines, the chronic loneliness these individuals experience can lead to an anti-depressant prescription for the patient. Nevertheless, the primary purpose of using these medications is to help lessen the symptom effects, encourage participation in therapy, and even help boost the prospects of engaging in activities. In conjunction with psychotherapy, individuals with SzPD should begin to show some improvement in their symptoms and have feelings of progress regarding their prognosis.

Despite the little research on SzPD and the infrequent encounters in clinical environments, there is a decent handle on how to treat it. However, there is still a concern regarding the typical patterns of SzPD. As prognosticated earlier, many people, even clinicians, see SzPD as one-size-fits-all. At least four of the seven criteria must be present, and it does not appear during the duration of a psychotic disorder or during another condition that has psychotic features, as outlined in the DSM (APA, 2013). With the presentation of atypical symptoms, misdiagnosis can occur, as the signs may not strictly adhere to DSM criteria. Presenting this way is not to say that they do not have SzPD. For example, if they attend a family gathering, they may entertain the children or do the cooking. Doing some sort of task prevents them from the realization of socialization. Sitting down and talking to people is a fear-based situation for these individuals, and their natural egosyntonic instinct is to avoid this feeling. Another example includes an individual with a regular job who takes their lunch away from other colleagues. They work with their colleagues but require this break from social interaction.

When strictly adhering to the criteria outlined in the DSM, these examples would violate those essential features. These individuals are doing something other than a solitary activity as they are participating in and being a part of a family. For the latter example, they are not working under isolated conditions, even if they show emotional detachment. However, when interpreting these situations, diagnosticians may say that these circumstances go against the hallmarks. Therefore, their ruling is that the patient does not have SzPD. However, the reality could be that they indeed do have SzPD and have now been misdiagnosed. The lack of research also plays a part here because thousands could share similar, atypical traits, but insufficient research has led to inadequate evidence.

Along comparable lines, individuals may present with schizoid traits, covert schizoid, or another co-occurring disorder, all of which can open the door for misdiagnoses or improper diagnoses. Schizoid traits are characteristics of the condition but are not enough to qualify for a complete SzPD diagnosis. Note that these traits may or may not be atypical, but they differ in terms of only being a few or a lesser severity than the full symptoms. Therefore, a patient may present with three schizoid traits of lower severity and an atypical feature, but this specific combination of criteria does not warrant a diagnosis. Covert schizoid presents as sociable and flexible in a way because these individuals mask their feelings. This masking allows them to fit in and appear normal but makes it much harder to diagnose and, more often than not, leads to a misdiagnosis. Lastly, when an equivalent or co-occurring disorder is present, there are increases in the likelihood of an improper diagnosis. The desire for isolation may be due to paranoid personality disorder. The appearance of emotional coldness could be due to obsessive–compulsive personality disorder. While these are just two examples, they are still highly plausible for being mistaken as SzPD. Yet, they can also be a comorbid condition. Therefore, clinicians must consider these other potential disorders when evaluating this disorder.

Another important topic to note is the underestimation of SzPD and schizoid traits with suicide. Studies show that SzPD, covert schizoid, and schizoid traits are major risk factors for completed suicides and serious attempts (Attademo et al., 2021). Isolation, loneliness, lack of close relationships, and emotional detachment are hallmarks of SzPD and are also significant factors for suicide. Once again, the lack of research on SzPD fails these individuals and now puts them at risk due to the underestimation. Clinicians must be aware of these traits and provide appropriate assessments to individuals closely resembling these signs. Care plans and treatment must also account for the patient's potential unwillingness to cooperate in this intervention.

The final topic of importance is the connection between SzPD and violence. Misconceptions arise regarding SzPD because many tie it to schizophrenia. However, this is another error in thinking because individuals with schizophrenia or SzPD are usually not violent. Patients with schizophrenia have a high likelihood of committing a violent crime, but this is primarily due to comorbid substance abuse (Cho et al., 2019). Therefore, with the proper management of this comorbid disorder and an understanding of specific risk factors, the prevention of violence and aggression can occur (Cho et al., 2019). It is important to note that violence can also occur as a result of inadequate management of schizophrenia (i.e., forgetting medications or missing therapy).

Nevertheless, individuals with schizoid do not generally show violent tendencies. Knowing the key characteristics of the disorder, the highest chance of violence arising stems from their emotions that cause disinhibition. The feelings of detachment, not finding pleasure in activities, and wanting to be alone open these individuals up to the possibility of impulsiveness, recklessness, and other self-destructive behaviors. Openness to new solitary experiences, such as using drugs in secrecy, can follow. Depending on the substance (i.e., marijuana, cocaine, et cetera) and the amount in question, the effects on the person can differ. The consequences of drugs have particular characteristics, but at the end of the day, they do affect people differently. Regardless of the effects, most drugs, including sedatives, increase the likelihood of aggressive behaviors. Research shows that those with drug use disorders have a four to ten times higher chance of committing a violent act (Zhong et al., 2020). Along with the forenamed impulsiveness, emotional dysregulation and the formation of delusions are additional risk factors for violence that are present in people with PDs (Howard, 2015).

Interestingly, research has found exceptions to the notion that schizoid is not a traditionally violent PD. A study on Greek prisoners found that violent crimes, attempted homicides, and completed homicides were significantly associated with Cluster A disorders of SzPD and schizotypal PD, even though a majority of the incarcerated individuals were diagnosed with a Cluster B disorder, mainly Antisocial PD (Apostolopoulos et al., 2018). The study also shows that serial offenders are more inclined to possess schizoid traits (Apostolopoulos et al., 2018). In addition to violence, these individuals are likely to engage in sexual fetishism, sexual masochism, exhibitionism, and voyeurism (Apostolopoulos et al., 2018). While it may seem to be a contrast to the criteria, remember that individuals with SzPD have a rare interest in having sexual experiences with others; that is not to say they cannot do or view things themselves that bring them gratification.

Other studies show that violent behavior increases with substance use disorders and SzPD, but still conclude that the majority of people with psychiatric disorders are not violent (Pulay et al., 2008). In a case study, a man attempted to kill his wife and kill himself but failed. The second time, he successfully killed his wife but was unsuccessful in committing suicide. Nine years later, when all appeared to be going well and with no concerns, he committed suicide. During previous stressful times, he had these ideations. The authors concluded that the violence against his wife and himself was the result of decompensation, or decline in illness manageability, of his SzPD (Loza & Hanna, 2006). Under periods of stress, this led to the decompensation of his SzPD (Loza & Hanna, 2006). Ultimately, this led to the development of a brief psychotic episode during the successful and unsuccessful attempts (Loza & Hanna, 2006).

These studies and examples further prove the need for more research regarding SzPD. The case study shows why there is an additional demand for emphasis on the causes of decompensation in SzPD. There is also a need for a supplemental investigation to mitigate this risk. SzPD is a riveting, complex, and relevant topic. These individuals come from all walks of life and live without much notice from others. Understanding this information and the misconceptions is crucial as there are wrong and hurtful associations and stereotypes to SzPD. As the facts hold, these individuals are not naturally violent. Their impulsive choices and the progression or regression of the disorder are the primary causes of this atypical behavior. While the misconceptions of violence are relevant to society today, it is still incredibly consequential to state that there is a vital need for more research on the diagnostics, treatment, and effects of SzPD.

3 Methods

In terms of methodology, the primary and sole method used was a literature review. For this composition of data, there was no limit to how long ago a publication date was. The reason for this was the sole fact that literature and findings are scarce concerning SzPD. Sources were collected using broad searches through PubMed and Google Scholar. The simple search term "Schizoid Personality Disorder" was used.

For more direct points, keywords such as "Misconceptions," "Violence," "Therapies," "Treatments," "Progression," "Traits," "Symptoms," or "Explanations" were used. There are many articles and sources out there that can provide information regarding SzPD. However, most of these articles reference the DSM or other scientific compositions in the first place. Therefore, going directly to the source allows for minute misinterpretation. Each of the selected articles had their abstracts reviewed first before referencing the results, discussion, or conclusion. Due to the lack of research, it was paramount to determine the validity and reliability of these articles. There was concern with finding and reporting on papers considered faulty or insufficient. However, after much analysis, it is believed that the academic and scientific articles and sources referenced above do not apply to this category. The omission of a few of these problematic articles occurred after resulting in the preliminary searches.

Additionally, many of these articles on SzPD build on another's findings, so this paper followed the same format. However, this paper opted to do things a little differently. In each section of importance, it was easier to incorporate minute discussions and insights to help minimize the potential for misinterpretation. The complexity of this information can easily cause one to get lost, so this approach was necessary for readability. Furthermore, the author consulted with Dr. Marina Bornovalova at the University of South Florida. This consultation was a discussion to gain further insight into the disorder, but the incorporation of that information into this paper did not transpire.

4 Discussion

Within this paper, the assessment of the most critical aspects of schizoid personality disorder took place. Based on the information presented here, the outcomes of SzPD can be favorable with proper diagnosis and treatment. For those who enter therapy, the future looks positive, considering the current psychotherapies and pharmacotherapies available. However, the presented information shows how much there is still to learn and research concerning this disorder. There is a need to know what demographics are more susceptible, alongside the true causes and risk factors. There is a need to explore new treatments and set up longitudinal studies to ensure that therapeutics and interventions for SzPD have been effective over the years. In addition, there is a need concerning the potential comorbid disorders and how to treat them, or how to prevent schizoid from progressing to a condition like schizotypal personality disorder. When the number of research articles increases, eventually, there will be a surge of quality research. More minds will get thinking and building, and more paths within this topic will diverge.

Along these lines, refinement to the current criteria can occur. SzPD is one-size-fits-all in the eyes of some, and will one day no longer have that view. This aspiration is another reason for the call for more investigation on this topic. With advancements in understanding, schizoid traits, atypical symptom presentation, and covert schizoid can be understood better. When these concepts are better acknowledged, the prevalence rates of attempted and complete suicide can decrease. It is this connection that also runs consecutively. Acceptable and reliable research provides the resources to grasp these poorly understood variations. Following this, proper and explicit identification of these variations increases while improper diagnoses or misdiagnoses can decrease ubiquity. By being aware of the signs and indications, clinicians can implement more suitable interventions. Achieving such a goal helps to minimize the chance of suicide and aids in reducing the possibility of aggressive behaviors and violence. Saving lives and protecting others is the primary outcome of conducting and implementing new research.

One interesting question arises when discussing the facts about SzPD. If the scientific community knows that individuals with SzPD do not seek help but are aware of the risks they face as a result, then why do they not choose to pursue answers that would better help these patients? Unfortunately, there is no clear answer to this question. The most logical conclusion is that there is hardly any research on this topic, and what is published does not call other researchers to action or inspire them to pursue new avenues. Therefore, the patients are left needing help, but help is hard to provide because a lack of strategies gained from research is absent.

There are indeed treatments available right now. The therapies and interventions are also effective. However, the first problem is that a limited number of treatment options are available, and sadly, they do not work for every patient who walks into the door. The second is that research is providing no new treatments. New treatments for depression and anxiety are undergoing experimentation nearly every day. The same applies to other conditions, such as schizophrenia. It is simply illogical not to investigate new treatments and therapies when research proves a need for novel interventions. A form of logical fallacy is present in this debate and requires a medical ethicist to provide input. While individuals with SzPD are egosyntonic and are usually happy with their lives, evidence shows that this maladaptive lifestyle results in substantial emotional harm. Not being able to derive pleasure from activities and not wanting to form relationships with people is heartbreaking. Now, think of how most people live and compare that to the hallmarks of SzPD. The realization is that these individuals are missing out on life. Life is different for everyone, but think of the highs, the lows, all the fun, or the unfortunate sadness. Think of living a life that is exciting or one with meaningful connections and true love. Instead, people with SzPD experience chronic loneliness and feel nothing about the outside world. Wanting to help give these individuals a true life should be motivating and encouraging enough to continue research into effective therapies.

5 Conclusion

After reviewing the selected literature, there is clear evidence that behavioral and therapeutic researchers need to focus more attention and time on SzPD. While the evidence has shown that individuals with SzPD do have emotional difficulties with their maladaptive behaviors, most lead a life they are happy with. However, other evidence shows that it is not wise to allow these individuals to remain in their current way of life for long. For example, it shows chronic loneliness that is unbearable and can lead to crippling depression. Depression can progress to a point where suicide appears to be the best option. Another example shows that severe stress can cause a psychotic break and can potentially lead to harming oneself or another. Observations show the same consequences with a comorbid substance use disorder. However, this condition exacerbates the potential for recklessness, self-deteriorating behavior, suicidality, and the harming of others. The cause of this is simply impulsiveness, which has its primary motivation due to the inability to regulate emotions. These examples show overwhelming support for needing proper diagnostic criteria, proven effective long-term treatment, techniques to reduce or eliminate risk factors, and strategies for diminishing the likelihood of comorbidities arising.

Some form of a schizoid personality has been around since the first edition of the DSM. To this day, there is still debate and controversy over whether it belongs in the DSM in the first place, whether it is a different form of avoidance attachment style, whether there is a need for a division into two distinct categories with one aiming more towards avoidant PD and one towards schizotypal PD, or whether cluster A PDs are simply different traits of a sole personality disorder. Nevertheless, the point here is that psychologists and researchers are spending more time debating the definition and classification of this disorder instead of trying to help the people affected by it. Those who are starting to develop the disorder need a comprehensive treatment plan to curb this disturbance before it gets out of hand. Those who are progressing through the condition need effective treatments and therapies before things escalate to harmful and damaging behaviors. The solutions and goals are within reach, but more effort is required to obtain them.

References

American Psychiatric Association. (2013). Diagnostic and statistical manual of mental disorders (5th Ed.). https://doi.org/10.1176/appi.books.9780890425596

Apostolopoulos, A., Michopoulos, I., Zachos, I., Emmanouil, R., Georgios, T., Vasiliki, M., Charalambos, P., & Athanasios, D. (2018). Association of schizoid and schizotypal personality disorder with violent crimes and homicides in Greek prisons. *Annals of General Psychiatry*. https://doi.org/10.1186/s12991-018-0204-4

Attademo, L., Bernardini, F., & Spatuzzi, R. (2021). Suicidality in individuals with schizoid personality disorder or traits: A clinical mini-review of a probably underestimated issue. *Psychiatria Danubina, 33*(3), 261–265. https://doi.org/10.24869/psyd.2021.261

Căndel, O.-S., & Constantin, T. (2017). Antisocial and schizoid personality disorder scales: Conceptual bases and preliminary findings. *Romanian Journal of Applied Psychology, 19*(1), 10–16.

Cho, W., Shin, W. S., An, I., Bang, M., Cho, D. Y., & Lee, S. H. (2019). Biological aspects of aggression and violence in Schizophrenia. *Clinical Psychopharmacology and Neuroscience: THe Official Scientific Journal of the Korean College of Neuropsychopharmacology, 17*(4), 475–486. https://doi.org/10.9758/cpn.2019.17.4.475

Cuijpers, P., Karyotaki, E., Ciharova, M., Miguel, C., Noma, H., & Furukawa, T. A. (2021). The effects of psychotherapies for depression on response, remission, reliable change, and deterioration: A meta-analysis. *Acta Psychiatrica Scandinavica, 144*(3), 288–299. https://doi.org/10.1111/acps.13335

Eaves, S., & Rey, J. A. (2016). Brexpiprazole (Rexulti): A new monotherapy for schizophrenia and adjunctive therapy for major depressive disorder. *P & t: A Peer-Reviewed Journal for Formulary Management, 41*(7), 418–422.

Esterberg, M. L., Goulding, S. M., & Walker, E. F. (2010). Cluster a personality disorders: Schizotypal, schizoid and paranoid personality disorders in childhood and adolescence. *Journal of Psychopathology and Behavioral Assessment, 32*(4), 515–528. https://doi.org/10.1007/s10862-010-9183-8

Fariba, K. A., Madhanagopal, N., & Gupta, V. (2022). Schizoid personality disorder. StatPearls Publishing. https://www.ncbi.nlm.nih.gov/books/NBK559234/

Frank, E., Novick, D., & Kupfer, D. J. (2005). Antidepressants and psychotherapy: A clinical research review. *Dialogues in Clinical Neuroscience, 7*(3), 263–272. https://doi.org/10.31887/DCNS.2005.7.3/efrank

Howard, R. (2015). Personality disorders and violence: what is the link? *Borderline Personality Disorder and Emotion Dysregulation.* https://doi.org/10.1186/s40479-015-0033-x

Kendler, K. S., Czajkowski, N., Tambs, K., Torgersen, S., Aggen, S. H., Neale, M. C., & Reichborn-Kjennerud, T. (2006). Dimensional representations of DSM-IV cluster A personality disorders in a population-based sample of Norwegian twins: A multivariate study. *Psychological Medicine, 36*(11), 1583–1591. https://doi.org/10.1017/S0033291706008609

Kendler, K. S., Myers, J., Torgersen, S., Neale, M. C., & Reichborn-Kjennerud, T. (2007). The heritability of cluster A personality disorders assessed by both personal interview and questionnaire. *Psychological Medicine, 37*(5), 655–665. https://doi.org/10.1017/S0033291706009755

Klonsky, E. D., Jane, J. S., Turkheimer, E., & Oltmanns, T. F. (2002). Gender role and personality disorders. *Journal of Personality Disorders, 16*(5), 464–476. https://doi.org/10.1521/pedi.16.5.464.22121

Koch, J., Modesitt, T., Palmer, M., Ward, S., Martin, B., Wyatt, R., & Thomas, C. (2016). Review of pharmacologic treatment in cluster A personality disorders. *The Mental Health Clinician, 6*(2), 75–81. https://doi.org/10.9740/mhc.2016.03.75

Loza, W., & Hanna, S. (2006). Is schizoid personality a forerunner of homicidal or suicidal behavior?: A case study. *International Journal of Offender Therapy and Comparative Criminology, 50*(3), 338–343. https://doi.org/10.1177/0306624X05285093

Martens, W. (2010). Schizoid personality disorder linked to unbearable and inescapable loneliness. *The European Journal of Psychiatry.* https://doi.org/10.4321/S0213-61632010000100005

Pulay, A. J., Dawson, D. A., Hasin, D. S., Goldstein, R. B., Ruan, W. J., Pickering, R. P., Huang, B., Chou, S. P., & Grant, B. F. (2008). Violent behavior and DSM-IV psychiatric disorders: Results from the national epidemiologic survey on alcohol and related conditions. *The Journal of Clinical Psychiatry, 69*(1), 12–22. https://doi.org/10.4088/jcp.v69n0103

Stone, M. (1993). Long-term outcome in personality disorders. *The British Journal of Psychiatry: THe Journal of Mental Science, 162*(3), 299–313. https://doi.org/10.1192/bjp.162.3.299

Tantam, D. (1988). Lifelong eccentricity and social isolation. II: Asperger's syndrome or schizoid personality disorder? *The British Journal of Psychiatry: THe Journal of Mental Science, 153*, 783–791. https://doi.org/10.1192/bjp.153.6.783

Winsper, C., Bilgin, A., Thompson, A., Marwaha, S., Chanen, A. M., Singh, S. P., Wang, A., & Furtado, V. (2020). The prevalence of personality disorders in the community: A global systematic review and meta-analysis. *The British Journal of Psychiatry: THe Journal of Mental Science, 216*(2), 69–78. https://doi.org/10.1192/bjp.2019.166

Zhong, S., Yu, R., & Fazel, S. (2020). Drug use disorders and violence: Associations with individual drug categories. *Epidemiologic Reviews, 42*(1), 103–116. https://doi.org/10.1093/epirev/mxaa006

Part IV

Case Studies and Solution-Based Interventions

Skipping Stones: Gaps in Syrian Humanitarian Aid

10

Natalie Nagib

Abstract

This chapter delves into the significant health disparities faced by Syrian women, particularly in the context of the ongoing conflict and the challenges within refugee camps. Despite global advancements in technology and health, the chapter highlights the persistent gap in health equity, exacerbated by social determinants that disadvantage vulnerable populations. The Syrian crisis has devastated the nation's infrastructure, with profound implications for women's health, especially in the areas of sexual and reproductive health, and mental well-being. This chapter examines challenges in humanitarian aid, including inadequate data collection and gender bias, which have left critical gaps in assistance. The discussion extends to the compounded challenges introduced by the COVID-19 pandemic, which has further strained the already limited resources available to refugees and internally displaced persons (IDPs). Through a detailed analysis, the chapter proposes immediate and long-term solutions, emphasizing the importance of culturally sensitive interventions and the active participation of affected communities to ensure sustainable outcomes. Ultimately, this chapter calls for a renewed focus on addressing the health needs of women in humanitarian crises, advocating for political stability as a foundation for effective aid and the eventual restoration of Syria's health and social systems. It underscores the critical role that women play in the peacebuilding process and the necessity of gender-sensitive policies in humanitarian efforts.

Note While this chapter specifically references women's challenges when discussing gender issues, it is important to point out that women are not the only group that faces gender issues, and it is imperative to include other groups such as LGBTQ+ in the conversation.

N. Nagib (✉)
Lake Erie College of Osteopathic Medicine, Bradenton, FL, USA
e-mail: nnagib62841@med.lecom.edu

S. Spowart (ed.), *Global Happiness and Humanitarian Assistance*, Integrated Science 29, https://doi.org/10.1007/978-3-031-71789-5_10

Keywords

Syrian women's health • Sexual and reproductive health • Mental health • Sexual violence against women in refugee camps

1 A Public Health Introduction

1.1 Health Disparities

With the technological developments, health advancements, and global wealth progress that define the twenty-first century, health inequities and disparities continue to rise, creating a larger gap between the wealthy and healthy, and the sick and disadvantaged. The social determinants of health help frame the conversations surrounding the historical role of global health inequities and disparities. While there is much research in the literature regarding the adverse effects of the social determinants of health and how many lives it impacts through international databases and independent scientific studies, there is a jarring gap in the literature. There is sufficient data to indicate that there is indeed a public health crisis presented globally as a result of the social determinants of health leading to health inequities and disparities. Unfortunately, the gap in literature lies in the field of study of actions that can be taken to rectify the damage, reduce disparities, close the gap, and attain health equity. This is especially true in the field of humanitarian assistance, where the scope of research is still dangerously narrow (Irwin et al., 2006; Krieger, 2014).

1.1.1 Gender as a Health Disparity

When discussing health inequities and disparities, it is vital to discuss the social determinants of health (SDOH) (Satcher, 2010). The SDOH can be grouped into five domains which affect the health outcomes of a person: economic stability, education access and quality, health care access and quality, neighborhood and built environment, and social and community context. In essence, a person's birthplace, where they grow up, live, work, and age, coupled with the health systems that are operating to deal with illness, all directly affect their health, even if unintentionally (U.S Department of Health and Human Services, Office of Disease Prevention and Health Promotion [ODPHP], n.d.). Unfortunately, these factors/SDOH are biased since their creation, based on the societal context they were founded in. These biases include racial, gender, age, disability, and religious discrimination- to list a few example- that systemically sideline and disadvantage certain populations and people within populations. When certain populations are institutionally discriminated against based on, for example, gender, nearly every social determinant of health works against their favor and places their health in a disadvantaged state (Penman-Aguilar et al., 2016). The issues are exacerbated if the systems in place to treat their illnesses are also biased and leave them to be exploited and die at higher rates than their counterparts. The discussion of disparities is extremely relevant and critical in the field of humanitarian assistance.

1.2 Humanitarian Assistance

Human-made disasters have resulted in some of the greatest humanitarian crises seen in history. Two notable human-made disasters are the conflicts in Syria and Yemen, both of which have been termed the world's largest humanitarian crisis (Alhaffar & Janos, 2021; NRC, 2019). These humanitarian crises began as conflicts and wars started by humans and resulted in catastrophic disasters claiming the lives of many civilians and military personnel. These deadly events lead to crises requiring humanitarian action and intervention to save the lives of those impacted by the incidents. Unfortunately, there exist gapping disparities in humanitarian aid which impact the health outcomes of a population experiencing a humanitarian crisis.

1.3 Syrian Humanitarian Crisis

This chapter will focus on the Syrian crisis and the way humanitarian aid has skipped stones leading to gaps in assistance. Unfortunately, the nature of the crisis has allowed for the vulnerabilities of women, especially refugee and internally displaced women, to be exploited and preyed on. This leads to worsening women's health, sexual and reproductive health, mental health, and increased sexual violence against women in this context. All of this has been exacerbated with the ongoing COVID-19 pandemic which has worsened the situation for all humanitarian contexts, especially for refugees and internally displaced populations (IDPs) who are congregated in congested camps and require specific aid. The situation in Syria, while plagued with its own set of circumstances, is not novel to the field of humanitarian assistance and the rest of the world. It is critical to consider this specific situation, propose and implement solutions, and provide important lessons for implementation in other existing and future problems in the global humanitarian field.

2 Background Information

2.1 Crisis in Syria

2.1.1 Pre-Crisis Era

The complexities of the Syrian crisis mirror the intricate array of players involved with underlying issues transcending the events of March 2011. Bashar al-Assad's authoritarian rule suppressed dissent and imprisoned critics during his leadership (Karim & Islam, 2017). Tight control over media and favoritism in economic policies marked his tenure, further stifling free speech and political expression (Aboultaif, 2016; Gürcan, 2020; Karim & Islam, 2017; Mirza et al., 2021). The nation's human rights record was notably bleak, upheld through familiar dictatorial tactics that stifled free speech and prohibited political expressions (Karim & Islam, 2017). Additionally, the deteriorating social and economic conditions are cited as contributing factors to the crisis's onset (Aboultaif, 2016; Gürcan, 2020; Karim & Islam, 2017; Mirza et al., 2021). Widespread unemployment and restricted access to essential necessities such as food, water, electricity, and medical supplies characterized the challenging circumstances (Karim & Islam, 2017; Musarurwa & Kaye, 2016). Over time, the proliferation of corruption fostered the emergence of a new affluent class spanning various religious affiliations (Karim & Islam, 2017).

Competing interests in gas and future energy extraction among Middle Eastern nations, Russia, and the US are believed to have played a role in exacerbating the Syrian crisis (Ghoble, 2015; Karim & Islam, 2017). Moreover, the water crisis in Syria acted as a catalyst for the violence that erupted in 2011 (Karim & Islam, 2017; Musarurwa & Kaye, 2016). A severe drought in 2006 inflicted significant devastation, impacting over 1.3 million people and leading to the loss of up to 85 percent of livestock in certain regions (Karim & Islam, 2017). The dire consequences forced residents from 160 villages to abandon their homes due to crop failures (Karim & Islam, 2017). Prolonged drought, accompanied by internal migration, poverty, and unemployment, created a socio-economic upheaval marked by water scarcity (Karim & Islam, 2017; Musarurwa & Kaye, 2016). The insufficient response from both the government and the international community in addressing this crisis further fueled violent protests against the government (Aboultaif, 2016; Gürcan, 2020; Karim & Islam, 2017; Mirza et al., 2021).

The arrest of children in Daraa, which sparked anti-government protests in Syria, was profoundly insensitive and widely condemned (Karim & Islam, 2017; Musarurwa & Kaye, 2016). With a police force consisting of only a few thousand officers, security forces lacking proper training in handling internal disturbances were deployed (Karim & Islam, 2017). Additionally, the Assad regime employed sectarian pro-regime militias, known as the Shabiha or "ghosts" in Arabic (Karim & Islam, 2017). These civilian militias were frequently dispatched to disrupt protests, resulting in the frequent killing of unarmed demonstrators (Karim & Islam, 2017). The use of excessive force in numerous instances further fueled widespread grievances among the populace (Aboultaif, 2016; Gürcan, 2020; Karim & Islam, 2017; Mirza et al., 2021).

2.1.2 History and Evolution of the Crisis

March of 2022 marked the eleventh year of the Syrian conflict that began in 2011 during the rise of the Arab Spring and has been described as the worst humanitarian crisis of the twenty-first century. The conflict has displaced 6 million Syrians internally, forced millions more out of the country, and hundreds of thousands have been killed, injured, disabled, and are unaccounted for. Major destruction was inflicted upon the infrastructure in the nation, including healthcare, education, social status, economic crisis, and has led to the largest need for humanitarian aid and assistance of this decade. This has had a significant impact on the health status of the Syrian population in Syria, who lack access to medical services due to the mass exodus of healthcare providers fleeing the conflict, straining the remaining facilities and personnel. The lack of primary health care services in Syria has reduced the health status of the entire nation and has forced millions of them to seek refuge in neighboring countries, such as Turkey (Alhaffar & Janos, 2021). The intense conflict which has resulted in several consequences and weakened the available resources, has demanded global attention and humanitarian assistance and relief (Alhaffar & Janos, 2021). Humanitarian aid has been focused on addressing the pressing concerns and needs of the population. This aid attempts to reach the 13.7 million Syrian who have been displaced, 6.7 million of which are internally (Mercy Corps, 2021).

2.1.3 COVID-19 Complexities

More than half of the nation's population requires assistance, which is equal to 11.1 million people (Reid, 2021). Of the refugee population, close to half are children under the age of 18, accounting for 2.5 million people in need (Mercy Corps, 2021). Additionally, 70% of the population lives below the poverty line, although this number has been steadily increasing as a result of the COVID-19 pandemic (United Nations High Commissioner for Refugees [UNHCR], 2021). There are 12.4 million people who are food insecure in Syria, and 1.3 million are severely food insecure (World Food Programme [WFP], 2021). As the COVID-19 pandemic evolves, Syrians are faced with two crises.

The pandemic has introduced added layers of complexity and challenges for the Syrian refugee population since they find themselves in contexts of poor water access, sanitation, and hygiene (WASH); overcrowded living quarters; and declining economic conditions (Mercy Corps, 2021). Additionally, the pandemic has disrupted the supply chain of medical equipment and cleaning supplies. While several refugees are receiving information to protect themselves from the virus, they lack the resources to be able to do so (Alhaffar & Janos, 2021). This has caused a weakened COVID-19 response and has added to the challenges already faced in the Syrian humanitarian crisis.

2.1.4 Consequences of the Crisis

After the many years of crisis in Syria, the long-term effects of war are being noticed including PTSD, life-long disability, and other downward trends in social and emotional well-being, in addition to physical wellness (Cheung et al., 2020). This at-risk population has been further impacted by the health disparities in the nation arising due to the inaccessibility of primary care facilities due to distance, reduced safety, diminished public transportation, or relocation of citizens (Kherallah et al., 2012). All of these factors force patients into positions that heighten their risk of illness, injury, disability, and death which define health disparities.

The Syrian conflict has evident negative impacts on the population's well-being and individual health. A study conducted found that the physical, mental, and social well-being of Syrians substantially declined as a result of the war. It was concluded that there were similar effects on well-being regardless of whether Syrians were directly or indirectly exposed to conflict. Participants were 3.57 times more likely to be dissatisfied with healthcare during the conflict as opposed to before the war. The prevalence of negative emotions among Syrians increased by 41.4.% during the conflict. This decline in health and well-being has been determined to be unparalleled in any other country worldwide, even those where war, protests, and disasters are being experienced in similar magnitudes (Cheung et al., 2020). Based on The World Happiness Report, between 2013 and 2019, the average happiness index for Syria was 3.39 points (with a low of 3.01 in 2015 and a high of 3.89 in 2013). This value was below the 5.42 global average in 2019 based on 153 countries (TheGlobalEconomy.com, n.d.). These staggering results highlight the critical nature of this public health crisis and the need to restore peace and well-being in Syria.

2.1.5 Intergenerational Consequences

The Syrian war has several short- and long-term effects on health and intergenerational consequences. The obvious short-term effects include physical traumas, health center closures, minimal health personnel, reduced accessibility, among others. As the war has ravaged the nation for several years, the long-term effects of the war are becoming increasingly evident including disability, mental health issues, intergenerational stress, and infrastructure destruction of the healthcare system in Syria. Long-term research following the civil war in Sierra Leone has demonstrated the intergenerational impacts of war on mental health and psychosocial well-being which can be extrapolated to the situation in Syria. Those who survive conflict are at higher risks for depression, anxiety, early life shocks, and posttraumatic stress disorder (Betancourt et al., 2020; Singhal, 2018). Additionally, these individuals are faced with family separation; lack of education, healthcare, food, and shelter; face a stigma; and experience loss of family and community acceptance. All these factors further contribute to the depleting mental state of war survivors (Al Ibraheem et al., 2017; Betancourt et al., 2020). Other long-term, intergenerational effects include chronic stress, malnutrition, disability, mental scars, and more (Devakumar et al., 2015; Their News team, 2018). The high prevalence and lasting effects of war on the individual and population health will cause further strain on the already diminished healthcare system that will require rebuilding while simultaneously draining the system.

While the entire population is suffering, there is a disproportionately negative effect on maternal and child health during the conflict in Syria. When the conflict first began, much of the interventions that were implemented by humanitarian organizations were focused on trauma care and infectious disease control (Akik et al., 2020). As a result, there was a significant decline in the quality of reproductive, maternal, newborn, child, and adolescent health and nutrition (RMNCAH&N) interventions. This skewed focus in aid has created a disparity for women's health which is a critical discussion within the context of the global humanitarian field.

3 The Gap: Impact on Women

3.1 Women's Health & Sexual and Reproductive Health

The war has claimed hundreds of thousands of lives and reduced the health status of the entire population (Cheung et al., 2020). Women's health and sexual and reproductive health (SRH) are no exception and have not been spared; rather the war has exacerbated the issue and gap in women's health status compared to the rest of the population (Akik et al., 2020). The war has resulted in direct and indirect effects on women's health including reduced access to healthcare and necessary services. This has reduced their quality of life through the lens of diminished health performance, reduced happiness, and discrimination in the foreign country they find themselves in. Several vital health indicators have demonstrated a decline in the health status of women and their SRH (Çöl et al., 2020). Food and water insecurity, poor sewage systems, inadequate vaccination, ecological challenges, overcrowded and unsanitary living quarters, are important risk factors that threaten the health status of the refugees and host community. Reproductive health services have also been cited as a service requiring special consideration and attention (Alhaffar & Janos, 2021).

3.2 The Impact in Numbers

One study conducted among Syrian women in a Turkish refugee camp found poor indicators of SRH. Among the participants, 51.3% married before the age of 18 years, which increased after the war and was associated with education and length of stay in the camp. Of the participants, 16% were pregnant, and of those, 26.7% did not receive prenatal care, 47.7% experienced a miscarriage, and 50.8% reported symptoms of sexually transmitted infections (STIs). Of those sexually active, 37.8% did not use a contraceptive. A third of women deliver with complications, and morbidity among Syrian infants is higher than Turkish (Samari, 2017). The study concluded that there was a need for reproductive health services and education (Şimşek et al., 2017).

Another study found that the influx of Syrian refugees in Turkey has resulted in higher rates of adolescent births, under 5-mortality, both of which were mediated by the increase of adolescent marriages among females under 18 years (Cinaroglu, 2021). An assessment of Syrian women's health in Turkey was conducted through the framework of Minimum Initial Service Package, MISP, which is an established set of minimum and priority reproductive health services to be activated and delivered at the onset of a humanitarian crisis (Çöl et al., 2020). The results found that 56% of marriages were consanguineous, and that adolescent marriage was very high. Antenatal care rate was inadequate, and only 20% of women had regular gynecological visits. Among married women, 24% used a modern contraceptive, and 35% had unmet family planning needs. Lastly, reports of sexual violence were around 8% (Çöl et al., 2020). Given the diminished infrastructure within Syria, it is challenging to find current and comprehensive health data of internally displaced women. In refugee camps, particularly in Turkey and Jordan as they host the largest number of Syrian refugees, data collection is slightly more streamlined in the camp setting, although still not ideal (Çöl et al., 2020).

3.3 Sexual Violence Against Women: Community & Familial Ostracization

To compound on the issue of declining women's health and sexual and reproductive health, Syrian women face increasing sexual violence both within the camp setting and externally. Several news reports and studies have discovered women are being sexually exploited in return for aid for themselves and their families (BBC, 2018). This form of exploitation also occurs in other host countries such as Turkey and Jordan, where women are seeking safety from their war in Syria, only to be met with sexual and gender-based violence (Ibesh et al., 2021; Roupetz et al., 2020; Samari, 2017). While there is strong evidence to demonstrate this increasingly projected violence against women, a substantial portion of the public literature on the response to the Syrian refugee crisis remains gender blind, despite the fact that organizations responding to the crisis are increasingly aware of the need to address their requirements (Rohwerder, 2018). Tragically, not only are women violated as they seek out aid and assistance, but they face rape and torture within prisons.

There have been an overwhelming number of personal accounts of violence against women within the prisons. For years, women were ashamed to speak out regarding the violence they endured in prisons due to the stigma and the culture. Those who were exhausted and wanted to be heard faced backlash from their families and communities. Some women were killed by their families due to the perceived shame brought upon them, while others were abandoned by their families and communities for being 'unclean'. This sort of response was brutalizing and victimizing these women over again, in addition to the original assault. Additionally, it was extremely scarring and traumatizing for these women to experience this level of hatred and disrespect (Al Jazeera English, 2014). The trauma endured by women, however, is not only physical and can manifest as mental health concerns.

3.4 Impacts on Mental Health

The war has resulted in direct and indirect effects on women's health including reduced access to healthcare and necessary services. This has reduced their quality of life through the lens of diminished health performance, reduced happiness, and discrimination in the foreign country they find themselves in. Syrian women refugees in Turkey have revealed negative experiences and unhappiness relating to the journey of motherhood in a foreign country (Korukcu et al., 2017). Additionally, Syrian women are taken as polygamist wives to Turkish men resulting in discrimination by the rest of Turkish society as they are viewed as adulterers (Duman, 2020). There is escalating gender-based violence against girls and women in the camps and due to economic disparities and hardship, Syrian women have turned to sex work. Beyond the physical and economic hardships, there is an emotional burden, 55% need psychological support (Samari, 2017). These negative experiences of discrimination and marginalization are internalized by women and impacts their mental health status.

3.5 Gaps in Aid and Discrimination

As mentioned earlier, there are gaps in aid which arise from many barriers and factors, such as discrimination. Turkey recognizes Syrians as "guests" and not refugees due to asylums only being granted to those from Europe. Thus, the millions of Syrians in Turkey are overcrowded into 22 government-run camps with limited support (Samari, 2017). While Turkey has introduced universal health care to its citizens and applied it to Syrians, it is not uniformly applied and 90% of refugees rely on the medical emergency stations and hospital tents on campsites. Those healthcare providers often face a language barrier and shortage of resources (Samari, 2017). Additionally, gender-based disparities exist as women's health-specific services were not implemented within an effective timeframe. The Minimum Initial Service Package (MISP) for Sexual and Reproductive Health in Crises was not initially implemented in Turkey, which lagged the services and responses, leading to an exacerbated issue presently for women's health.

3.5.1 Discrimination and the Disaster Data

Gender issues and disparities are critically important to recognize in every setting, but especially in humanitarian assistance since women (and other marginalized populations) face a unique set of challenges that require specific actions and considerations to address them. There is a recurring theme in the literature: when disaster strikes, men and women are not affected in the same way. Women are further victimized as they already face diminished economic and educational opportunities in their day-to-day life which are exacerbated at the onset of a disaster since it is harder for them to fend for themselves given the state that society has limited them to. There is gender data bias from everyday examples of car crash dummies being built for men to early warning systems favoring men over women. As society becomes desensitized to these disparities and considers it normal, less pressure is put into changing this tendency to ensure equality and equity in general and in their resilience to natural hazards. This is dangerous trend and cycle to enter that must be broken in order to ensure equity within the global humanitarian field. Current work being done by the World Health Organization varies from LGBTQ + health, equitable health systems, gender-responsive health systems, closing the data gender gap, and more. There are specific guidelines for gender-sensitive disaster management that need to be actively practiced in the field.

4 Current Challenges in the Field

4.1 Aid and Limited Disaster Data

Humanitarian assistance as a field aims to provide services and resources to those faced with a crisis, war, natural disaster, among other incidents. It is an important field of work that faces several key challenges and issues which limit its success. While humanitarian help is increasing, it is doing so at a considerably slower rate than in the past (Urquhart, 2019). Aid flows must be expanded since crises are lasting longer and requiring more resources because they disproportionately affect the poorest and most vulnerable people (Urquhart, 2019). This is especially true in the context of the Syrian crisis which has severely impacted the economic standing of the nation.

As the conflict has disrupted and destroyed infrastructure in the region, it has led to limited disaster data and increased the challenge of healthcare and humanitarian aid delivery in Syria (Alhaffar & Janos, 2021). As mentioned earlier there is also the gender disparity in disaster data that is an additional challenge that needs to be addressed. While technological advancements and public engagement have sped up and improved the supply of aid, there are still obstacles in this imperfect process. Disaster data has improved the delivery of help and the efficacy of humanitarian aid. Improved information systems have expanded disaster data over the last 25 years, but standardized data gathering has proven to be a problem (Walker & Walter, 2000). A research approach to address this challenge would determine an effective way to standardize disaster data collection through analysis of previous data collection methods that have been reliable and are replicable. When organizations are better able to track the magnitude of a problem and need, it allows for their efforts to be concentrated and effective in order to meet the health needs of refugee and displaced populations.

4.2 Resiliency and Self-Sufficiency

One of the most pressing problems of humanitarian aid is assuring the impacted people's resilience and self-sufficiency, so that when these organizations pull out, the local group can continue their own efforts and restore/rebuild their community. Future interventions and approaches should focus on resiliency and self-sufficiency training in humanitarian field work and how to best disseminate the information in the high stress environments of a crisis. When refugee and displaced populations are able to continue their aid and relief they will sustainably grow and overcome a crisis, improving the entire population's health.

5 Lessons Learned from Previous Aid

While many nations and organizations have provided varying forms of relief to Syria and its population, there has been a large inability to come up with a clear, effective response to stop the dismay of the millions of displaced people. Researchers, humanitarian agencies, local non-governmental organizations, and host governments need to pursue a new strategy that combines short-term emergency humanitarian aid and longer-term promises of development, sustainability, and dignity that come with economic and residential opportunities. As a result, both displaced persons and host communities will benefit and improve their status (Al Hussein, 2018). Solutions and programs must be culturally sustainable. It is also vital that the community is involved and can carry it out on their own and bolsters their livelihood and stimulates their economy. Moving forward, humanitarian relief should address the disproportionate effect of the war on women and children's health by concentrating new programs in this sector (Akik et al., 2020). Several organizations have called attention to the gap in women and children's health and call for funding and support in this area (Women for Women International, n.d.). Furthermore, there are rising concerns over the mental health of the population which require new interventions (Cheung et al., 2020). These lessons provide the foundations for recommendations for assistance and relief provided moving forward.

Through personal knowledge and cultural changes within the community, one health education delivered to Syrian refugee women in their own language was shown to have a substantial impact on women's understanding of their health and influenced their attitudes and motives (Erenoğlu & Yaman Sözbir, 2019). This emphasizes the necessity of accounting and confronting language, cultural, and religious obstacles in these populations' camps. According to another study, merely offering free services does not solve the problem; there are other cultural, linguistic, and traumatic variables at play that must be addressed (Inci et al., 2020). A program based on educational home visits was also shown to help women prepare for birth and lower the incidence of cesarean procedures (Doyle et al., 2014). Prenatal and antenatal care, according to another research, should be free, integrated into the community, cost-effective, provide information for patients and families, give inexpensive treatment alternatives, be prepared for issues, and have the expertise to refer to other particular specialties (Zanconato et al., 2006).

6 Proposed Solutions

6.1 Addressing the Immediate Needs of Women & Current Challenges in the Field

While there are pressing needs to continue to provide resources and essential services on the ground, the transition to long-term solutions and attention to women's and children's health must begin. As discussed, there are a variety of vulnerable populations that are further victimized and impacted by a crisis, especially when it requires them to be displaced and put into camps. Among these vulnerable populations are women. They face a unique set of challenges and as a result, it is critical to be prepared with certain accommodations and programs for these populations. Since there are immediate needs that are required at the onset of a crisis, the proposed accommodations and programs listed below will focus on those initial necessities first. This is not an exhaustive list as there are needs that require attention in the recovery and reconstruction phases as well.

6.1.1 Mental Health Resiliency Training

Building resilience is an important lesson from prior case studies, however, the literature has also called for a gendered approach to building resilience. There is a gender-disparity in the field of humanitarian assistance. Often, women have a harder time establishing credibility in foreign settings, particularly, patriarchal societies (Gritti, 2015). Additionally, women face greater risks and incidences of sexual harassment and gender discriminations, as well as a threat to their safety and security (Gritti, 2015). Women also are challenged with maintaining work-life balance in which they tend to have more familial responsibilities compared to their male counterparts (Gritti, 2015). Recognizing gender inequalities, acquiring gender-sensitive data, and incorporating these results into care practices are all important stages in improving community resilience. The care practices need to be completely customized and tailored to meet the needs of the Syrian women refugees.

In emergency response and humanitarian practice, multi-tiered public health services that span current health, community, education, social welfare, and other sectors must be developed and evaluated (Jordans & Tol, 2012). While significant strides have been made to improve the mental health status of affected populations, there are several paradigms that are often competing, and thus there is an urgent need for consensus for discussion, policy development, and policy implementation (Ventevogel, 2018). Lastly, developing resilience should not be viewed just as a personal issue, implying that it should be limited to the development of individual abilities, but rather as a communal issue that should be tackled in a more systemic and ecological manner (Gritti, 2015). There is a vital need for communal culture change and shift to ensure these gendered care practices and resilience building are implemented in a sensitive and appropriate manner.

6.1.2 Educational Intervention

An important proposed solution that has gained slow traction in practice and in the field are educational programs and interventions. In this particular context of sexual health education, the proposal is geared towards healthcare professionals, as well as both men and women as it is viewed as a couple decision. In broad terms, this education will encompass types of contraception; where it is available; how to use them; what services and screenings are available; who provides these services; and providing special consideration to adolescent girls. Additionally, it

Table 1 Immediate needs and examples for addressing women's health in disaster and refugee settings

Immediate needs	Examples
Identify specific needs of women	Food, water, maternal requirements, sanitary products, gynecological care, etc., further explored below
Ensure that emergency relief supplies include women's specific requirements	Sanitary products, contraceptive, underwear, baby food/formula, nutritional supplements, culturally appropriate clothing, toiletries, etc
Ensure women's access to sufficient and adequate food	Culturally specific Pregnant and breastfeeding women's specific needs Consult women on food items considered essential in aid packages
Aid distribution for women should be handled by women	Especially in conservative cultures, a diverse response team, including women is critical
Ensure that women's menstrual needs are met	Handled and distributed by women response teams
Ensure women's access to adequate toilet and bathing facilities	Vital for women's reproductive health Sanitary products/toiletries Water sources should be sufficient & reachable/accessible, safe from violence, separate from the men's toilets
Ensure women's access to free health care services	Comprehensive health services including gynecological, prenatal, antenatal care, etc Readily available and accessible/close proximity Adequate ratio of providers to patients Female care providers on staff
Ensure security and safety of women	Women committees of officers/security that rotate to monitor security and safety Female police/armed personnel as protective details at the camp Night security Training to ensure women raise concerns and seek assistance when needed
Protect women from violence and abuse	Similar to the security measures above with additional free legal services, medical examinations, reporting procedures, support groups, vigilant groups, improved lighting in the camp, etc
Ensure access to psycho-social counseling	Free services in response to the trauma with female professionals on staff

(continued)

Table 1 (continued)

Ensure women's participation in management of camps and temporary shelters	Women in leadership and decision-making roles in the camp Participate and share their knowledge and ideas Ensure their participation and safety by not having meetings in the evening/after dark
Ensure women's equal access to compensation payments and rehabilitation measures	Establish positions where women can achieve economic opportunities Women access and right to government/organization assistance themselves and not through male relatives who may abuse the payments for their own leisure
Ensure women's access to information on relief and rehabilitation measures	Camp wide meetings to share information Individual outreach/meetings to reach women Diverse team, representative of women being served
Raising women's awareness of their human rights	Mobilizing and empowering women to advocate for their human rights
Reach out to widows and women headed households	Ask about their needs Inquire about beliefs for appropriate response/aid Gain their insight, ideas, and suggestions

Note The examples are created for the context of women's reproductive and sexual health in Syria adapted from initial necessities cited by Gomez (2006)

is important to combat gender-based violence by creating safe spaces for women; breaking down stigmas; increasing mental health care; and Increasing security.

The proposal for educational programming and intervention for healthcare professionals will be centered on cultural competency and sensitivity when interacting with Syrian refugee patients. It will also increase knowledge and awareness of services they can refer their patients to in order to increase use of family planning services and gynecological visits. This will provide a channel to disseminate information and services to patients and address some of the barriers and factors that preclude health service seeking behaviors such as mistrust of healthcare professionals and cultural barriers. These intensive training sessions can range from a few sessions within a week, or extended to a month or more, based on access and feasibility of the program.

The second aspect of the proposed program deals with direct outreach to the patients and their families to provide information regarding gynecological, obstetric, and family planning visits and what they entail including their benefits. Further discussions will cover the risks of not utilizing these essential healthcare services. The importance of employing family planning services and gynecological visits in the interest of the child and mother's health (and to preserve the mother's health for her existing children and family as well) will be highlighted. There is a great emphasis on family and the role of maternal figures in the household in regard to caring for their children and families, and thus framing the conversation and discussion in this light is critical (West et al., 2016). The program will also cover health literacy and agency to enable health service seeking behavior and how all family members can be involved in this process. The length of this phase would range from six months to one year, based on feasibility, as behavioral interventions necessitate rapport building and great time commitments to achieve desired outcomes.

Another important target audience of the program are men in the community, since women explain that it is their spouses who typically have the final say in the decisions (West et al., 2016). Educating men is vital to ensure women are empowered by their husbands to seek these services and promote their health. The setting for these conversations can be at religious gatherings and provided by other men/prominent religious leaders to receive their approval and increase buy-in of the community. Furthermore, these presentations can be provided at their job sites/work in the form of informational seminars and questions and answers (Q&A) discussions/panels. This style will foster conversation and dialogue to address concerns and questions of community members. In order to be effective and culturally relevant, educational interventions must be conducted in the refugees' native language (Arabic) and include members of the community/population.

It is equally important to address the cultural aspect of family planning and fertility among young couples/younger generations of refugees since there is tremendous stress put on them by older generations for procreation (West et al., 2016). Starting the conversation regarding this at younger ages in school through presentations and eventually having it a part of the curriculum can start the conversation early and begin to change the culture surrounding SRH. Children/youth are more impressionable than older generations in the community, allowing the program to take a proactive approach of informing and equipping them with the necessary knowledge to take charge of their health care for themselves. The school setting allows for streamlined outreach and simplified regulation given the structured setting. Additionally, students will be among their peers allowing for a comfortable environment. As previously stated, the strong focus on family and the maternal role in the home will be used to frame the dialogue and discussion. It will also be delivered in a linguistically appropriate manner (native tongue of Arabic) and culturally appropriate by members of the community.

This training technique is unique in that it focuses on the social factors that predispose, reinforce, and enable women in the target group to seek healthcare. The educational program will focus on a dual-layer model to educate healthcare practitioners and women's families. Healthcare providers will be educated on cultural competence and sensitivity, as well as cognizant of referral services for their patients. The second layer is to educate males and children in the community to shift cultural norms and enable women to seek family planning services and utilize gynecological care to ameliorate their health outcomes, for everyone's benefit. Furthermore, because women's health impacts the entire community, it moves the burden from women to equally spread it throughout the population. The program aims to influence people's cultural attitudes and social circumstances in order to achieve realistic behavior change. It is crucial in fostering women's sexual and reproductive health agency in order to increase their overall health, happiness, and quality of life in addition to defending their human right to health. This educational program's success would set a precedent for future culturally sensitive and long-term implementation among other refugee communities in settlements across the world.

6.2 Women Empowerment and Presence in the Camps

Women's voices and concerns need to be heard and their presence at the table is important. Not only should they be physically there, but they should play active roles that engage, enable, and empower them to gain a sense of control and power in their lives and decisions pertaining to their safety and health.

Conflict is experienced differently by men and women and even though women may not directly engage as combatants, they suffer greatly. Both the causes and the aftermath of wars are gendered, and women are purposefully excluded from formal peace conversations. Humanitarian work and efforts to rebuild conflict-torn countries fails to take into account the circumstances and specific necessities of women. Notwithstanding, women at the grassroots level are able to actively engage in peacebuilding and rehabilitation of their communities. In Syria specifically, women have not only survived but made substantial efforts for peace. It is critical to critically challenge the narrative that describes women as only a group with unique needs and requirements, and instead view them as proponents for peace and resiliency. In Syria, women have made inspiring headway in the rehabilitation of housing, food, health, work and financial security, changed roles, isolation, and gender-based violence. Their roles in all of these spheres are shaping new narratives for women, peace, and security that are distinct from the prevalent ones (Asaf, 2017).

In this context, women's empowerment intertwines with cultural and religious contexts, necessitating a nuanced approach that respects and integrates diverse beliefs and societal norms. Contrary to misconceptions, empowering women significantly contributes to societal stability by fostering inclusive growth, elevating education levels, improving healthcare access, and diversifying perspectives within communities, thereby strengthening the social fabric and enhancing overall resilience (Galiè, 2013; Wyler, 2020). It is important that humanitarian aid research understands why there is resistance and how to address it or adapt the solution to satisfy as many stakeholders as possible. This research would reduce the barriers in solution implementation to move long-term solutions from theory to practice. This would finally achieve a state of existence where humanitarian aid will not be a pressing issue globally, but rather solutions exist to end decades of crises and improve the health of refugees and displaced populations.

6.3 Policy Implementation

Unfortunately, there are not any substantial policies or regulations implanted in order to address the pressing issue of SRH of Syrian refugee women in Turkey and other refugee settlements globally. While this is troubling for women currently, it provides the opportunity for development and proposal of effective, meaningful, and purposeful policies and regulations to address this gap. This can be seen as a facilitator of the health program since there are no obvious limitations imposed, however, this also means there is no support either. Another consideration is the political tension of providing aid to refugees who are viewed as 'foreigners.' The political optics of the situation may hinder/impede the success of proposed solutions. Additionally, evidence-based policies for disaster data are necessary to aid in closing the gender disparity in disaster data and the humanitarian field. Furthermore, for comprehensive mitigation and bridging disparities, sexual violence mitigation policies are necessary.

6.3.1 Sexual Violence Mitigation Policy

A particular study which involved 55 Syrian and South Sudanese refugee women and girls took on an innovative and ethnographic approach to gathering data on sexual exploration and abuse (SEA) experiences while receiving humanitarian aid for themselves and their peers. Data collection included methods of reflection, action analysis, sketching, theater, storytelling, community mapping, and body mapping. SEA was found in all types of humanitarian aid investigated, and these findings were used to change how aid is distributed (Potts et al., 2022). When working with impacted populations, including refugees who face barriers such as illiteracy (as well as technological illiteracy) and lack of training may be overcome through the use of creative and participatory techniques, allowing for increased

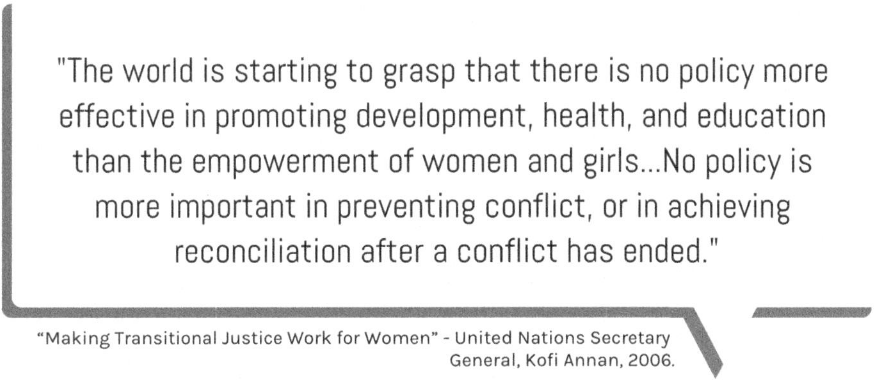

Fig. 1 Quote from Kofi Annan on the empowerment of women in transitional justice

co-production of information and evidence (Potts et al., 2022). This can be translated into practice to make aid delivery safer and policy implementation to protect women.

6.4 Long-Term Political Solution

The political dimension of the situation demands the resolution of political tensions via public health policy. Weapon-free zones, which provide a safe haven for individuals to reside and get medical care, should be expanded as part of the approach. There are few small areas where residents can seek refuge, which is exacerbated by the fact that the rest of the nation is either war torn or occupied by adversaries. The expansion of weapon-free zones across Syria's war-torn country would eventually lead to a cease-fire between all conflict sides. From here, policies for repairing the nation's and people's health status and outcomes may be developed and implemented. The next phase will be to reestablish the education sector and other specialized health programs before integrating long-term care for the war's aftermath. It is critical that the measures be implemented in this order, as these solutions will crumble if the conflict does not cease. According to the UN Secretary-General, there is only a political solution to this issue, not a military one (Guterres, 2020). Because the Syrian crisis is political, not military, the parties to the conflict must strive toward a cease-fire after establishing a series of weapon-free zones to permit democratic conversation and political settlement (Bennis, 2014). Any attempt to address other aspects of the Syrian situation without stopping the conflict would be ineffective since international humanitarian law violations have gone unpunished (Omar, 2020). The frequency of attacks on medical institutions has remained stable in recent years, indicating that international violators are not being held accountable for using healthcare facilities as a weapon of war. As a result, emphasis of activism for this health concern should be political stability. This will afford Syrians hope and the opportunity at a prosperous future through international accountability and support. Following the establishment of peace, the nation and its people will have a sense of direction. Syria, Syrian allies, and aid agencies will be able to offer medical assistance as well as work on rebuilding and restoring the country in all impacted areas, without abandoning any citizens (Martineau et al., 2017).

6.5 Sustainability and Funding

As mentioned earlier, one of the most important considerations in the success of humanitarian projects is the sustainability of the assistance. It is necessary that the intervention is implemented at a grassroots level- engaging the local community- and is able to be continued when the aid organization withdraws. In crises that are long-term without a definitive end, such as the case of the Syrian crisis, this fact is paramount. It is vital that the community members are able to pursue the project and that funding is sustainable. Ideally, these projects will not merely pump resources into the community, but rather, stimulate economic activity and generate jobs and income opportunities in the target community. In such ways, not only is the community benefitting from a public health standpoint, but from an economic view as well. This will help address the sustainability and funding of project, which are often the reasons for 'failed' attempts in the field. It is critical that the planning process account for a long-term implementation strategy to ensure success of efforts.

7 Conclusion: Next Steps

7.1 In Short

This chapter explored the Syrian crisis specifically relating to the issue of gender disparities and gaps in humanitarian aid. It explored the discrimination against female refugees and IDPs (Internally Displaced Populations) relating to mental health, women's health, and SRH (Sexual and Reproductive Health), and sexual violence. It provided some evidence-based interventions based on the literature including education, policy implementation, and immediate interventions that can be implemented in camps to support women during the transition period.

7.1.1 The Educational Step Forward

As discussed in the 'Proposed Solutions: Educational Intervention', the suggested educational training approach is unique in its innovation because it targets the social elements that predispose, reinforce, and empower women to seek health-care among the target population. Additionally, it shifts the burden from women to equitably distribute it across the community since women's health affects the entire community. For realistic behavior change, the program is intended to modify cultural beliefs and social factors around people, rather than pressuring the individual to change. This program is critical in promoting women's agency over their sexual and reproductive health in order to improve their overall health, happiness, and quality of life. The success of this educational program would set a precedent for future culturally sensitive and long-term implementation among other refugee populations in settlements around the world.

7.1.2 The Political Step Forward

As explored in the 'Proposed Solutions: Long-term Political Solution', the ten-year battle has demonstrated that none of the band-aid remedies attempted previously are long-term or viable since they do not address the underlying problem. Because the war is still political at its root, the solution must be political rather than military. Expansion of weapon-free zones and calls for an eventual cease-fire offer Syrians safe locations to seek sanctuary and necessary services. It is critical to find a solution as soon as possible to handle the issue in order to avoid losing any more generations to the conflict and to advance Syria toward restoration, which includes all citizens.

As the Syrian crisis closes on its ten-year anniversary, the effects of the war on infrastructure, healthcare systems, but most importantly the health, well-being, and livelihood of Syrians is catastrophic and has not gone unnoticed. Several organizations and nations have been pumping in millions of dollars of resources into the aid and relief of the population, however, there are still gaps and challenges that remain in this temporary solution. Lessons learned have shown that humanitarian aid and assistance must take on a long-term outlook and be culturally appropriate. It is vital for the sustainability of these efforts that community members are directly involved in the provision of these activities to not only increase their hope, livelihood, and dignity, but to also begin the process of transitioning to normalcy with a stimulated economy. Targeted response to support women not only improves the health of women and their children, but also impacts the greater community since women play a vital role in their respective communities. Additionally, improving the health of women allows for the protection and defense of their human rights.

References

Aboultaif, E. W. (2016). Regional and International factors that prolong the Syrian Crisis. *Syria Studies, 8*(2), 1–11.

Akik, C., Semaan, A., Shaker-Berbari, L., Jamaluddine, Z., Saad, G. E., Lopes, K., Constantin, J., Ekzayez, A., Singh, N. S., Blanchet, K., DeJong, J., & Ghattas, H. (2020). Responding to health needs of women, children and adolescents within Syria during conflict: Intervention coverage, challenges and adaptations. *Conflict and Health.* https://doi.org/10.1186/s13031-020-00263-3

Al Jazeera English. (2014). *Syrian women break their silence on rape. Al Jazeera English.* Retrieved June 10, 2022, from https://www.youtube.com/watch?v=93pH1ienj4U

Al Hussein, N. (2018). Foreword: Syria in 2018-in search of solutions. *Forced Migration Review, 1*(57), 4.

Al Ibraheem, B., Kira, I. A., Aljakoub, J., & Al Ibraheem, A. (2017). The health effect of the Syrian conflict on IDPs and refugees. *Peace and Conflict Journal of Peace Psychology, 23*(2), 140–152.

Alhaffar, M. H., & Janos, S. (2021). Public health consequences after ten years of the Syrian crisis: A literature review. *Globalization and Health.* https://doi.org/10.1186/s12992-021-00762-9

Asaf, Y. (2017). Syrian women and the Refugee Crisis: Surviving the conflict, building peace, and taking new gender roles. *Social Sciences, 6*(3), 110. https://doi.org/10.3390/socsci6030110

BBC. (2018). *Syria conflict: Women 'sexually exploited in return for aid'—BBC News. BBC News.* Retrieved June 10, 2022, from https://www.bbc.com/news/world-middle-east-43206297

Bennis, P. (2014, May 28). *5 Concrete Steps the US Can Take to End the Syria Crisis.* Transnational Institute. https://www.tni.org/es/node/13186

Betancourt, T. S., Keegan, K., Farrar, J., & Brennan, R. T. (2020). The intergenerational impact of war on mental health and psychosocial wellbeing: lessons from the longitudinal study of war-affected youth in Sierra Leone. *Conflict and Health.* https://doi.org/10.1186/s13031-020-00308-7

Cheung, F., Kube, A., Tay, L., Diener, E., Jackson, J. J., Lucas, R. E., Ni, M. Y., & Leung, G. M. (2020). The impact of the Syrian conflict on population well-being. *Nature Communications.* https://doi.org/10.1038/s41467-020-17369-0

Cinaroglu, S. (2021). The effect of increases in the Syrian refugee population in Turkey on public maternal and child health outcomes. *Health Care for Women International.* https://doi.org/10.1080/07399332.2020.1842411

Çöl, M., Bilgili Aykut, N., Usturalı Mut, A. N., Koçak, C., Uzun, S. U., Akın, A., Say, L., & Kobeissi, L. (2020). Sexual and reproductive health of Syrian refugee women in Turkey: A scoping review within the framework of the MISP objectives. *Reproductive Health*. https://doi.org/10.1186/s12978-020-00948-1

Mercy Corps. (2021, March 15). *The facts: What you need to know about the Syria Crisis*. Mercy Corps. Retrieved November 25, 2021, from https://www.mercycorps.org/blog/quick-facts-syria-crisis

Devakumar, D., Birch, M., Rubenstein, L. S., Osrin, D., Sondorp, E., & Wells, J. C. K. (2015). Child health in Syria: Recognising the lasting effects of warfare on health. *Conflict and Health*. https://doi.org/10.1186/s13031-015-0061-6

Doyle, O., McGlanaghy, E., Palamaro-Munsell, E., & McAuliffe, F. M. (2014). Home based educational intervention to improve perinatal outcomes for a disadvantaged community: A randomised control trial. *European Journal of Obstetrics Gynecology and Reproductive Biology, 180*, 162–167. https://doi.org/10.1016/j.ejogrb.2014.06.006

Duman, T. (2020). The situation of Syrian women in Turkey. *Comparative Demography of the Syrian Diaspora European and Middle Eastern Destinations*. https://doi.org/10.1007/978-3-030-24451-4_5

Erenoğlu, R., & Yaman Sözbir, Ş. (2019). The effect of health education given to Syrian refugee women in their own language on awareness of breast and cervical cancer, in Turkey: A randomized controlled trial. *Journal of Cancer Education, 35*(2), 241–247. https://doi.org/10.1007/s13187-019-01604-4

Galiè, A. (2013). Empowering women farmers: The case of participatory plant breeding in ten Syrian households. *Frontiers A Journal of Women Studies, 34*(1), 58–92.

Ghoble, V. T. (2015). Making of Syrian Crisis: The energy factor. *International Studies, 52*(1–4), 38–52.

Gomez, S. (2006). *Guidelines for gender sensitive disaster management: Practical steps to ensure women's needs are met and women's human rights are respected and protected*. Asia Pacific Forum on Women, Law and Development.

Gritti, A. (2015). Building aid workers' resilience: Why a gendered approach is needed. *Gender Development, 23*(3), 449–462. https://doi.org/10.1080/13552074.2015.1095542

Gürcan, E. C. (2020). Domestic and external factors in the Syrian conflict: Toward a multi-causal explanation. *The Regional Order in the Gulf Region and the Middle East: Regional Rivalries and Security Alliances, 331–350*, 1.

Guterres, A. (2020, February 21). *Syria | UN news*. United Nations. https://news.un.org/en/focus/syria

Ibesh, R., Ahmad, W., Chikhou, R., Jumah, R., Sankar, H., & Thurston, A. (2021). The educational experiences of Syrian women in countries of Safety/Asylum. *International Journal of Educational Research Open, 2*, 100027. https://doi.org/10.1016/j.ijedro.2020.100027

Inci, M. G., Kutschke, N., Nasser, S., Alavi, S., Abels, I., Kurmeyer, C., & Sehouli, J. (2020). Unmet family planning needs among female refugees and asylum seekers in Germany—is free access to family planning services enough? results of a cross-sectional study. *Reproductive Health*. https://doi.org/10.1186/s12978-020-00962-3

Irwin, A., Valentine, N., Brown, C., Loewenson, R., Solar, O., Brown, H., Vega, J. (2006, May 23). The commission on social determinants of health: Tackling the social roots of health inequities. PLOS Medicine. https://journals.plos.org/plosmedicine/article?id=10.1371%2Fjournal.pmed.0030106

Jordans, M. J., & Tol, W. A. (2012). Mental health in humanitarian settings: Shifting focus to care systems. *International Health, 5*(1), 9–10. https://doi.org/10.1093/inthealth/ihs005

Karim, S., & Islam, N. M. (2017). Syrian crisis: Geopolitics and implications. *Biiss Journal, 37*(2), 1.

Kherallah, M., Alahfez, T., Sahloul, Z., Eddin, K. D., & Jamil, G. (2012). Health Care in Syria before and during the crisis. *Avicenna Journal of Medicine, 2*(03), 51–53. https://doi.org/10.4103/2231-0770.102275

Korukcu, O., Aydın, R., Conway, J., & Kukulu, K. (2017). Motherhood in the Shade of migration: A qualitative study of the experience of Syrian refugee mothers living in Turkey. *Nursing Health Sciences, 20*(1), 46–53. https://doi.org/10.1111/nhs.12379

Krieger, N. (2014). Discrimination and health inequities. SAGE Journals. https://journals.sagepub.com/doi/https://doi.org/10.2190/HS.44.4.b?url_ver=Z39.88-2003&rfr_id=ori%3Arid%3Acrossref.org&rfr_dat=cr_pub++0pubmed

Making Transitional Justice Work for Women, https://www.unwomen.org/sites/default/files/Headquarters/Media/Publications/UNIFEM/0701_MakingTransitionalJusticeWorkForWomen_en.pdf

Martineau, T., McPake, B., Theobald, S., Raven, J., Ensor, T., Fustukian, S., Ssengooba, F., Chirwa, Y., Sreytouch, V., Wurie, H., Hooton, N., & Witter, S. (2017). Leaving no one behind: Lessons on rebuilding health systems in conflict- and crisis-affected states. *BMJ Global Health*. https://doi.org/10.1136/bmjgh-2017-000327

Mirza, M. N., Abbas, H., & Qaisrani, I. H. (2021). Anatomizing Syrian crisis: Enumerating actors, motivations, and their strategies (2011–2019). *Liberal Arts Social Sciences International Journal, 5*(1), 1.

Musarurwa, H. J., & Kaye, S. B. (2016). Unpacking the Syrian crisis: A literature review. *Information Management and Business Review, 8*(6), 32–38.

NRC. (2019, February 25). *Yemen: The man-made disaster must end*. Norwegian Refugee Council. Retrieved December 1, 2021, from https://www.nrc.no/news/2019/february/yementhe-man-made-disaster-must-end/

Omar, A. (2020). Understanding and preventing attacks on health facilities during armed conflict in Syria. *Risk Management and Healthcare Policy, 13*, 191–203. https://doi.org/10.2147/rmhp.s237256

Penman-Aguilar, A., Talih, M., Huang, D., Moonesinghe, R., Bouye, K., & Beckles, G. (2016). *Measurement of health Disparities, Health INEQUITIES, and social determinants of health to support the advancement of Health Equity*. https://www.ncbi.nlm.nih.gov/pmc/articles/PMC5845853/

Potts, A., Fattal, L., & Kolli, H. (2022). Engaging refugee women and girls as experts: Co-creating evidence on sexual exploitation and abuse in humanitarian crises using creative, participatory methods. *Evidence Policy*. https://doi.org/10.1332/174426421x16420949265777

Reid, K. (2021, July 13). *Syrian refugee crisis: Facts, FAQs, and how to help*. World Vision. Retrieved November 25, 2021, from https://www.worldvision.org/refugees-news-stories/syrian-refugee-crisis-facts

Rohwerder, B. (2018, July 5). *Syrian refugee women, girls, and people with disabilities in Turkey*. OpenDocs Home. Retrieved June 10, 2022, from https://opendocs.ids.ac.uk/opendocs/handle/20.500.12413/13950

Roupetz, S., Garbern, S., Michael, S., Bergquist, H., Glaesmer, H., & Bartels, S. A. (2020). Continuum of sexual and gender-based violence risks among Syrian refugee women and girls in Lebanon. *BMC Women's Health*. https://doi.org/10.1186/s12905-020-01009-2

Samari, G. (2017). Syrian refugee women's health in Lebanon, Turkey, and Jordan and recommendations for improved practice. *World Medical & Health Policy, 9*(2), 255–274. https://doi.org/10.1002/wmh3.231

Satcher, D. (2010). Include a social determinants of health approach to reduce health inequities. *SAGE Journal*. https://doi.org/10.1177/00333549101250S402

Şimşek, Z., Yentur Doni, N., Gül Hilali, N., & Yildirimkaya, G. (2017). A community-based survey on Syrian Refugee Women's Health and its predictors in şanliurfa Turkey. *Women and Health, 58*(6), 617–631. https://doi.org/10.1080/03630242.2017.1321609

Singhal, S. (2018). Early life shocks and mental health: The long-term effect of war in Vietnam. *Journal of Development Economics*. https://www.sciencedirect.com/science/article/pii/S0304387818302268

Syria happiness index—data, Chart. TheGlobalEconomy.com. (n.d.). Retrieved June 24, 2022, from https://www.theglobaleconomy.com/Syria/happiness/

Their News team. (2018, March 15). *Seven ways that seven years of Syrian war has affected children and their education*. Their News. https://theirworld.org/news/seven-years-of-syria-conflict-how-it-affects-children-education-refugees-schools

U.S. Department of Health and Human Services, Office of Disease Prevention and Health Promotion. *Social Determinants of Health*. Social Determinants of Health—Healthy People 2030. https://health.gov/healthypeople/objectives-and-data/social-determinants-health

UNHCR. (2021). *Syrian refugee crisis: Aid, Statistics and News: USA FOR UNHCR*. Retrieved November 25, 2021, from https://www.unrefugees.org/emergencies/syria/

Urquhart, A. (2019, August 06). 4 trends in global humanitarian aid. Retrieved September 9, 2021, from https://www.bond.org.uk/news/2019/08/4-trends-in-global-humanitarian-aid#fig1

Ventevogel, P. (2018). Interventions for mental health and psychosocial support in complex humanitarian emergencies: Moving towards consensus in policy and action? *Mental Health of Refugee and Conflict-Affected Populations*. https://doi.org/10.1007/978-3-319-97046-2_8

Walker, P., & Walter, J. (2000). World disasters report 2000. The International Federation of Red Cross and Red Crescent Societies.

West, L., Isotta-Day, H., Ba-Break, M., & Morgan, R. (2016). Factors in use of family planning services by Syrian women in a refugee camp in Jordan. *Journal of Family Planning and Reproductive Health Care, 43*(2), 96–102. https://doi.org/10.1136/jfprhc-2014-101026

WFP. (2021). *Syrian Arab republic: World food programme*. UN World Food Programme. Retrieved November 24, 2021, from https://www.wfp.org/countries/Syrian-Arab-Republic?utm_source=google&utm_medium=cpc&utm_campaign=11625191502&utm_content=110051062221&gclid=EAIaIQobChMI_vjEy_mX9AIVlKXICh3bTQ5HEAAYASAAEgJHDvD_BwE&gclsrc=aw.ds

Women for Women International. (n.d.). *Conflict response fund: Support needed now*. Women for Women International. Retrieved November 26, 2021, from https://support.womenforwomen.org/crf-syria?src=GSCR21103A&ms=cpc_google_crf%2Bsyria&utm_medium=cpc&utm_source=google&utm_campaign=crf%2Bsyria&utm_content=gs-ad&gclid=EAIaIQobChMIwovu-IyY9AIVgajICh0gqw-aEAAYBCAAEgLXM_D_BwE

Wyler, C. (2020). *Keepers of the Cultural Flame: Women and the Role They Play in Maintaining and Nurturing Cultural Identity Within Refugee and Displaced Populations* (Doctoral dissertation, Nova Southeastern University).

Zanconato, G., Msolomba, R., Guarenti, L., & Franchi, M. (2006). Antenatal care in developing countries: The need for a tailored model. *Seminars in Fetal and Neonatal Medicine, 11*(1), 15–20. https://doi.org/10.1016/j.siny.2005.10.002

Beyond the Bell Curve: Positive Outliers

11

Nicole Nagib

Abstract

This chapter explores the concept of positive outliers in global health, defined as regions or countries that achieve superior health outcomes despite challenging conditions. It examines the multifaceted factors that characterize these outliers, including health indicators, social determinants of health, health system performance, innovative health initiatives, disease eradication efforts, and public health preparedness. By analyzing these cases, the chapter identifies key success factors and strategies that have led to positive health achievements. It also delves into how incentives, such as behavior change rewards, healthcare access support, and worker motivation, drive success in global health practices. Furthermore, the chapter discusses the ethical considerations surrounding profit in humanitarian crises and highlights successful global health initiatives, emphasizing the importance of multilateral partnerships, innovation, data-driven decision-making, and equity. The insights drawn offer valuable lessons for policymakers, public health practitioners, and global health stakeholders aiming to replicate these successful models to improve health outcomes worldwide.

Keywords

Positive outliers • Success • Incentives • Humanitarian initiatives • Global health

N. Nagib (✉)
University of South Florida, Tampa Campus, Tampa, FL, USA
e-mail: nicolenagib@usf.edu

S. Spowart (ed.), *Global Happiness and Humanitarian Assistance*, Integrated Science 29, https://doi.org/10.1007/978-3-031-71789-5_11

1 An Introduction to Positive Outliers in Global Health

A positive outlier within the landscape of global health signifies a distinct case, region, or country demonstrating notably superior health outcomes or extraordinary health-related accomplishments compared to the prevailing standards observed across many nations or regions worldwide. In statistical contexts, an outlier represents an observation significantly departing from the average or median within a dataset. In the realm of global health, a positive outlier emerges as an entity that surpasses established norms in a notably beneficial manner.

2 Factors that Characterize Positive Outliers

There are a variety of factors and metrics that can be used to quantify and characterize positive outliers in global health including health indicators, social determinants of health, health system performance, health initiatives and policies, disease eradication, and public health preparedness to name a few.

2.1 Health Indicators

Health indicators serve as crucial metrics in evaluating and characterizing positive outliers within the domain of public health. These indicators encompass a diverse array of quantitative and qualitative measures, such as mortality rates, life expectancy, disease prevalence, healthcare access, and socio-economic determinants of health (Pan American Health Organization [PAHO] & World Health Organization [WHO], n.d.). They provide a comprehensive snapshot of a population's health status and the effectiveness of health interventions. When identifying positive outliers, health indicators play a pivotal role by highlighting regions, communities, or countries that significantly surpass expected benchmarks or exhibit remarkably superior health outcomes compared to their counterparts (PAHO & WHO, n.d.). For instance, a positive outlier might showcase exceptionally low mortality rates from preventable diseases, notably high life expectancies, or innovative healthcare systems that ensure widespread access to quality care. By leveraging these indicators, public health practitioners can discern patterns, trends, and successful strategies that contribute to these exceptional outcomes. Moreover, the analysis of positive outliers enables the identification and dissemination of best practices and innovative approaches, fostering a deeper understanding of what drives exemplary health outcomes and offering valuable insights for global health policy formulation and implementation (PAHO & WHO, n.d.).

2.2 Social Determinants of Health

Social determinants of health play a pivotal role in characterizing positive outliers within the spectrum of public health. Positive outliers in social determinants of health denote regions or communities that exhibit exceptionally favorable socio-economic conditions, which significantly contribute to superior health outcomes (WHO, n.d.; WHO Commission on Social Determinants of Health, 2008). These outliers showcase robust social support systems, equitable access to education, stable employment opportunities, secure housing, and strong community cohesion, all of which play a crucial role in fostering overall health and well-being. By examining these positive outliers, public health experts gain valuable insights into the correlation between socio-economic factors and health outcomes (WHO, n.d.; WHO Commission on Social Determinants of Health, 2008). Understanding the success stories of regions where social determinants are notably favorable enables the identification and dissemination of strategies that address social inequalities and uplift communities, ultimately informing policies and interventions aimed at mitigating health disparities globally (WHO, n.d.; WHO Commission on Social Determinants of Health, 2008). Furthermore, the study of positive outliers in social determinants of health serves as a catalyst for advocating for policies that prioritize social equity, emphasizing the significance of addressing broader socio-economic factors in promoting better public health outcomes universally (WHO, n.d.; WHO Commission on Social Determinants of Health, 2008).

2.3 Health System Performance

Assessing health system performance serves as a pivotal tool in characterizing positive outliers within the realm of public health. A well-functioning health system encompasses various elements, including accessibility, quality of care, efficiency, equity, and responsiveness to the population's needs. Positive outliers in health system performance often manifest as regions or countries demonstrating exceptional efficiency in healthcare delivery, equitable access to services, and remarkable outcomes compared to global standards (Murray & Frenk, 2000). These outliers might showcase innovative approaches, robust infrastructure, effective policies, or streamlined healthcare delivery models that result in superior health outcomes (Murray & Frenk, 2000). By analyzing these positive outliers in health system performance, policymakers and public health experts gain invaluable insights into successful strategies and interventions that contribute to superior healthcare delivery (Murray & Frenk, 2000). Understanding the drivers behind these exceptional performances allows for the dissemination of best practices, facilitates cross-country learning, and informs the development of evidence-based policies aimed at enhancing health system resilience, equity, and effectiveness worldwide (Murray & Frenk, 2000). Additionally, recognizing and studying positive outliers in health system performance can inspire collaborative efforts to replicate and adapt successful approaches, ultimately contributing to advancing global health and achieving more equitable and efficient healthcare systems universally (Murray & Frenk, 2000).

2.4 Health Initiatives and Policies

Health initiatives and policies serve as instrumental benchmarks in characterizing positive outliers within the landscape of public health. These initiatives encompass a wide spectrum, including preventive programs, healthcare policies, community interventions, and public health campaigns aimed at addressing specific health challenges. Positive outliers often emerge in regions or countries where innovative, evidence-based health initiatives or policies have yielded exceptional outcomes, surpassing global norms or expectations (Schorr et al., 2014). These outliers might showcase groundbreaking interventions that effectively reduce disease burden, promote healthier lifestyles, enhance healthcare access, or address social determinants of health in a comprehensive manner. By scrutinizing these positive outliers in health initiatives and policies, policymakers and public health practitioners gain invaluable insights into successful strategies, impactful interventions, and policy frameworks that significantly contribute to improved health outcomes (Schorr et al., 2014). This analysis facilitates the identification and dissemination of best practices, encourages knowledge-sharing among nations, and informs the development of adaptable, context-specific policies and interventions globally. Furthermore, studying and learning from these positive outliers can inspire collaborative efforts to replicate successful initiatives, fostering a collective drive toward achieving better public health outcomes worldwide.

2.5 Disease Eradication

Disease eradication represents the pinnacle of success in public health, and its role in characterizing positive outliers is profound. Positive outliers in disease eradication signify regions or countries that have achieved extraordinary success in eliminating specific diseases or significantly reducing their prevalence to levels substantially lower than the global average (Centers for Disease Control and Prevention [CDC], 1999). These outliers often demonstrate exemplary strategies involving comprehensive vaccination campaigns, robust surveillance systems, effective healthcare infrastructure, and community engagement. Instances of positive outliers in disease eradication, such as the eradication of smallpox or near-elimination of diseases like polio in certain regions, exemplify exceptional dedication, innovation, and collaboration among healthcare stakeholders (CDC, 1999). By examining these positive outliers, public health experts can glean valuable insights into successful eradication strategies, enabling the identification and dissemination of best practices, innovative approaches, and the development of adaptable frameworks applicable to diverse global contexts. Additionally, the study of disease eradication outliers fosters international collaboration, encourages resource sharing, and catalyzes collective efforts aimed at replicating successful strategies, ultimately advancing the global agenda towards disease elimination and improving public health outcomes worldwide.

2.6 Public Health Preparedness

Public health preparedness constitutes a critical aspect of characterizing positive outliers in the realm of public health. Positive outliers in public health preparedness are exemplified by regions or countries that showcase exceptional readiness and resilience in confronting health emergencies, disasters, or pandemics. These outliers exhibit robust healthcare infrastructure, efficient response systems, well-defined emergency protocols, and proactive planning that significantly surpasses global standards. They demonstrate the ability to swiftly detect, respond to, and mitigate health threats while minimizing their impact on communities (Clements & Casani, 2016). Analyzing these positive outliers in public health preparedness provides valuable insights into successful strategies, innovative approaches, and effective interventions that enhance readiness and response capacities (Clements & Casani, 2016). By studying these cases, policymakers and health authorities can identify and disseminate best practices, facilitate international cooperation, and bolster global efforts to strengthen preparedness and response mechanisms (Clements & Casani, 2016). Furthermore, the examination of positive outliers in public health preparedness encourages collaborative learning and the implementation of adaptive strategies, contributing to more resilient and responsive public health systems worldwide (Clements & Casani, 2016).

3 In Summary: Factors that Characterize Positive Outliers

Positive outliers within global health represent invaluable case studies that offer profound insights and lessons for nations and regions worldwide. These exceptional instances serve as reservoirs of knowledge, unveiling key success factors and methodologies that hold the potential to elevate health outcomes on a broader scale. Delving into the intricacies of these outliers allows for the identification of best practices, innovative strategies, and effective interventions that can be adapted and tailored to diverse contexts. However, it is imperative to acknowledge the nuanced nature of each country or region, recognizing that while certain strategies may offer inspiration, their direct applicability might vary due to contextual disparities. Hence, while learning from positive outliers is immensely beneficial, it is crucial to exercise caution and consider the unique socio-cultural, economic, and healthcare landscape of different settings when implementing or transferring strategies for optimizing global health outcomes.

4 Defining Success in Global Health Initiatives

Defining success within the realm of global health initiatives necessitates a comprehensive assessment of multifaceted factors shaping the overall impact and efficacy of the program. Success, in this context, manifests through diverse indicators and outcomes that mirror the initiative's core objectives and its capacity to enhance the health and welfare of the intended population. Several pivotal considerations emerge when discerning success in global health initiatives. These encompass a spectrum of facets such as the initiative's alignment with set goals, its ability to drive positive health outcomes, its sustainability, community engagement, equity in access, cost-effectiveness, and adaptability within varying socio-cultural contexts. Evaluating success through these lenses provides a holistic understanding of an initiative's effectiveness and its enduring impact on global health paradigms.

5 Factors Used to Determine Success in Global Health Initiatives

When assessing success in global health initiatives, yet again, several factors and quantifiers may be employed such as health outcomes, equity and accessibility, cost-effectiveness, sustainability, capacity-building community engagement, and adaptability, among a handful of possible metrics.

5.1 Health Outcomes

Health outcomes stand as pivotal benchmarks when delineating success within the realm of global health initiatives. These outcomes encompass a spectrum of measurable indicators, including reduced mortality rates, increased life expectancy, diminished disease prevalence, improved maternal and child health, enhanced access to healthcare services, and better overall well-being among targeted populations (Banati & Moatti, 2008). The efficacy of a global health initiative is often gauged by its ability to tangibly improve these health outcomes within the intended communities or regions. For instance, successful initiatives might demonstrate a marked decline in infectious disease transmission, lowered infant mortality rates, or increased vaccination coverage, all indicative of positive health advancements (Banati & Moatti, 2008). These tangible improvements not only signify the initiative's effectiveness but also signify its capacity to make substantial, sustainable differences in the lives of those it aims to serve (Banati & Moatti, 2008). Consequently, health outcomes serve as fundamental measurements in defining the success and impact of global health initiatives, reflecting their ability to effectuate tangible and lasting improvements in population health.

5.2 Equity and Accessibility

Equity and accessibility serve as fundamental pillars when defining success within the realm of global health initiatives. A successful initiative ensures equitable access to healthcare services and interventions, regardless of socio-economic status, geographical location, ethnicity, or other determinants (World Economic Forum, 2023). Achieving equity involves addressing disparities in healthcare access and outcomes, ensuring that marginalized or underserved populations receive the same quality of care as others (Braveman et al., 2011). Success in global health initiatives is measured not only by the overall health improvements but also by the degree to which it diminishes health disparities and enhances accessibility for vulnerable groups (Braveman et al., 2011). A truly successful initiative demonstrates a narrowing of health gaps among different populations, thereby promoting inclusivity and fairness in healthcare delivery (World Economic Forum, 2023). The equitable distribution of resources, coupled with increased accessibility to essential healthcare services, signifies the success of a global health initiative in its mission to improve health outcomes for all, leaving no one behind.

5.3 Cost-Effectiveness

Cost-effectiveness stands as a critical parameter in defining the success of global health initiatives, delineating the optimal allocation of resources to achieve maximum health impact. A successful initiative demonstrates efficient utilization of available funds and resources, ensuring that interventions deliver substantial health benefits at justifiable costs (CDC, 2021). Assessing cost-effectiveness involves evaluating the initiative's ability to achieve desired health outcomes while minimizing expenses, thereby maximizing the reach and impact of interventions. Initiatives that demonstrate high cost-effectiveness ensure that limited resources are utilized judiciously, maximizing their potential to benefit a larger population (Pierson & Verguet, 2023). Such initiatives often prioritize interventions that yield significant health improvements relative to their costs, enabling sustainable and scalable approaches that can be implemented across diverse settings (CDC, 2021). Ultimately, success in global health initiatives considers not only the magnitude of health improvements achieved but also the efficiency with which these improvements are attained in relation to the resources expended.

5.4 Sustainability

Sustainability stands as a pivotal criterion in defining the success of global health initiatives, encompassing the durability and long-term impact of interventions beyond their initial implementation. A successful initiative is characterized by its ability to engender enduring health improvements and maintain positive outcomes even after the conclusion of the program (Yang et al., 2010). It involves building resilient healthcare systems, fostering community engagement, and ensuring the continuous availability of resources necessary for sustained progress. Sustainability in global health initiatives entails integrating interventions within existing infrastructures, empowering local communities to take ownership, and fostering partnerships that endure beyond the initiative's lifespan (Yang et al., 2010). Achieving sustainability ensures that the gains made in health outcomes persist, creating a lasting legacy of improved health and well-being for the target population, thus exemplifying the success of the initiative in creating meaningful and long-lasting positive change.

5.5 Capacity-Building

Capacity-building is integral to the success of global health initiatives, emphasizing the empowerment and improvement of local systems, expertise, and infrastructure. Beyond immediate health outcomes, successful initiatives strengthen healthcare systems and communities by fostering knowledge transfer, skill development, and institutional fortification for sustainable improvements in healthcare delivery (Brown et al., 2001). Such initiatives prioritize nurturing a cadre of trained healthcare professionals and fortifying healthcare infrastructure to effectively address present and future health challenges. Through investments in capacity-building, global health initiatives establish a foundation for self-sufficiency, enabling communities to independently address their health needs, fostering resilience, and ensuring continued progress and enhanced health outcomes beyond the initiative's timeline (Brown et al., 2001). Therefore, capacity-building stands as a pivotal element in defining the success of global health initiatives, empowering communities and healthcare systems to thrive and adapt in evolving health landscapes.

5.6 Community Engagement

Community engagement constitutes a fundamental element in defining the success of global health initiatives, emphasizing the active involvement, and participation of communities in the design, implementation, and sustainability of health interventions. A successful initiative embodies a collaborative approach that values and integrates the voices, needs, and insights of local communities into every stage of the intervention process (Durrance et al., 2022). Meaningful community engagement ensures that initiatives are culturally sensitive, contextually relevant, and accepted by the communities they aim to serve, thus fostering trust and ownership (Haldane et al., 2019). Successful initiatives leverage community engagement to mobilize resources, build social capital, and promote health-seeking behaviors. They empower communities to become active partners in decision-making processes, encouraging the co-creation of solutions that address their unique health challenges (Durrance et al., 2022). By fostering a sense of ownership and fostering meaningful participation, community engagement becomes a hallmark of success in global health initiatives, ensuring interventions are more sustainable, impactful, and responsive to the diverse needs of the populations they serve.

5.7 Adaptability

Adaptability stands as a crucial determinant when defining the success of global health initiatives, highlighting the capacity of interventions to flexibly respond and evolve in dynamic and diverse contexts. A successful initiative demonstrates a proactive and agile approach, capable of adjusting strategies, methodologies, and interventions to suit varying cultural, social, and environmental conditions. It embodies the ability to learn from ongoing evaluations, feedback mechanisms, and changing circumstances, enabling timely modifications that enhance effectiveness and relevance (Abimbola & Topp, 2018). Initiatives that exhibit adaptability harness innovation and embrace evidence-based practices while remaining open to incorporating local insights and emerging technologies (Abimbola & Topp, 2018). The capacity to adapt ensures that interventions remain responsive to evolving health challenges, emerging threats, and shifting community needs, thereby maximizing their impact and sustainability. Hence, adaptability emerges as a critical characteristic in defining the success of global health initiatives, ensuring their relevance, efficacy, and long-term viability in an ever-changing landscape.

6 Incentives Used in Global Health Practices

In global health practices, incentives serve as multifaceted tools employed to stimulate specific behaviors, actions, or outcomes that harmonize with the overarching objectives of enhancing public health on a global scale and tackling prevalent health challenges worldwide. These incentives, strategically implemented, span diverse levels encompassing individuals, communities, healthcare providers, and governments. Their deployment varies, targeting various stakeholders to drive desired changes in health-related behaviors, improve healthcare delivery, foster innovation, and bolster policy implementation. Understanding the diverse applications of incentives in global health practices elucidates their pivotal role in incentivizing positive actions and fostering a conducive environment for sustainable health improvements across different strata of society and governance structures.

6.1 Health Behavior Change

In the realm of health behavior change, incentives play a pivotal role in encouraging and reinforcing positive health behaviors among individuals or communities.

Various incentives, both monetary and non-monetary, serve as motivators to prompt and sustain healthy actions (The Commonwealth Fund, n.d.). Financial rewards, such as cash incentives or reimbursements, or non-monetary incentives like gift cards, vouchers, or access to certain services, are employed to incentivize individuals to participate in preventive health measures (The Commonwealth Fund, n.d.). For instance, individuals might receive incentives for getting vaccinated against prevalent diseases, attending routine health screenings for early detection of health issues, or adopting healthier lifestyles like quitting smoking, increasing physical activity, or adhering to prescribed medications. These incentives serve as tangible acknowledgments for individuals' efforts towards prioritizing their health, potentially increasing compliance with health recommendations and fostering long-term positive behaviors (The Commonwealth Fund, n.d.). However, while incentives can effectively motivate behavior change, careful consideration should be given to their design to ensure they promote equitable access and do not inadvertently create disparities among different socio-economic groups. Moreover, the sustainability and long-term impact of these incentivized behaviors should also be taken into account to ensure lasting health improvements.

6.2 Healthcare Access and Utilization

In resource-limited or underserved settings, incentivizing healthcare access and utilization can significantly impact the health outcomes of marginalized populations. Incentives are employed to address barriers that hinder individuals or communities from accessing essential healthcare services. For instance, transportation allowances or subsidies on healthcare costs are effective incentives that help alleviate financial burdens and logistical constraints for marginalized populations (Abduljawad & Al-Assaf, 2011). By providing financial support for transportation expenses or subsidizing healthcare costs, individuals who might otherwise face economic or geographical obstacles can more readily access medical facilities, consultations, treatments, and necessary medications (Abduljawad & Al-Assaf, 2011). These incentives act as facilitators, encouraging individuals to seek timely medical care, attend appointments, and engage in preventive health measures, consequently enhancing healthcare utilization among underserved communities (Abduljawad & Al-Assaf, 2011). However, it is crucial to ensure that such incentives are designed and implemented in a manner that prioritizes the needs of the most vulnerable groups, fostering equitable access to healthcare services without creating additional disparities (Abduljawad & Al-Assaf, 2011). Sustainable funding and monitoring mechanisms are also vital to ensure the continued availability and effectiveness of these incentives in promoting improved healthcare access and utilization for marginalized populations.

6.3 Health Worker Motivation

In the context of healthcare worker motivation, incentives serve as crucial tools to bolster the morale, retention, and performance of healthcare professionals, especially in underserved areas or during public health crises. These incentives are tailored to recognize and reinforce the dedication and efforts of healthcare workers operating in challenging environments (Abduljawad & Al-Assaf, 2011). Performance-based bonuses, salary enhancements, and financial rewards are common incentives used to acknowledge exceptional work, encourage high-quality service delivery, and recognize achievements in meeting healthcare goals or targets (Abduljawad & Al-Assaf, 2011). Additionally, offering training opportunities, continuing education programs, or career advancement prospects helps healthcare workers improve their skills, enhance job satisfaction, and feel valued within their profession (Abduljawad & Al-Assaf, 2011). Improved working conditions, including access to necessary equipment, supportive supervision, and a conducive work environment, are also crucial incentives that contribute to healthcare workers' motivation and overall well-being (Abduljawad & Al-Assaf, 2011). These incentives not only acknowledge the dedication of healthcare workers but also aim to alleviate burnout, retain skilled professionals in underserved areas, and strengthen the healthcare workforce's resilience during public health emergencies. However, the effectiveness of these incentives depends on their alignment with the needs and preferences of healthcare workers, and sustainable implementation is vital to ensure long-term motivation and retention within the healthcare workforce.

6.4 Research and Innovation

In the realm of research and innovation within global health, incentives serve as catalysts driving scientific breakthroughs and advancements. Funding agencies, governmental bodies, philanthropic organizations, and research institutions utilize incentives to inspire and support researchers, scientists, and entrepreneurs in developing novel solutions to address pressing health challenges. These incentives take various forms, such as research grants, prizes, awards, or competitive funding opportunities, provided to individuals or teams undertaking innovative projects. They incentivize the pursuit of cutting-edge medical technologies, new drug discoveries, diagnostic tools, or interventions aimed at combatting specific health issues. By offering financial support or recognition through grants, prizes, or awards, incentives encourage creativity, risk-taking, and collaboration among researchers, ultimately fostering the development of impactful solutions (Cooper, 2016). Moreover, these incentives facilitate the translation of scientific discoveries into practical applications, accelerating the pace of innovation and driving the creation of interventions that can significantly impact global health outcomes. However, the sustainability and continued availability of funding, coupled with mechanisms for fair distribution and equitable access to research opportunities, are crucial to ensuring that incentives effectively stimulate ongoing research and innovation in global health.

6.5 Public Health Campaigns

Incentives play a pivotal role in driving participation and achieving desired outcomes in public health campaigns, especially during vaccination drives or disease control programs. To encourage engagement and compliance with health targets, communities are often offered incentives that serve as motivational rewards for their active involvement (Glanz, 1997). These incentives can take various forms, including food rations, educational materials, community development projects, or other tangible benefits. For instance, communities may receive food aid or supplementary nutrition for meeting vaccination coverage goals, attending health education sessions, or actively participating in disease control initiatives. Educational materials such as books, pamphlets, or workshops may be provided to promote health literacy and awareness. Additionally, community development projects like infrastructure improvements or access to clean water might be offered as incentives, fostering a sense of community ownership and demonstrating the long-term benefits of active participation in public health endeavors. These incentives not only motivate communities to actively engage in health-promoting behaviors but also contribute to fostering a sense of empowerment, community mobilization, and sustained involvement in ongoing public health initiatives. However, it is crucial to ensure that the incentives offered are culturally appropriate, sensitive to local needs, and do not inadvertently create dependencies or perpetuate inequalities within communities. Sustainable and transparent distribution mechanisms are also imperative to uphold the effectiveness and integrity of such incentive-based public health campaigns.

6.6 Public–Private Partnerships

In the domain of global health, incentives serve as instrumental tools in fostering collaborative efforts between public and private sectors through incentivizing public–private partnerships. Governments often utilize incentives to encourage private sector involvement in developing and delivering healthcare services, innovative technologies, or interventions aimed at addressing health challenges. One common incentive provided by governments to entice private sector engagement is offering tax breaks, subsidies, or other financial incentives. These incentives create an environment conducive to collaboration by reducing financial burdens and incentivizing private entities to invest in healthcare research, infrastructure development, or service provision. For instance, tax incentives might be offered to pharmaceutical companies to spur research and development of vaccines or treatments for neglected diseases (Trouiller et al., 2002). Additionally, financial benefits could be extended to private healthcare providers to expand their services to underserved areas or to invest in healthcare technologies. By leveraging incentives, governments aim to stimulate innovation, improve healthcare access, and bridge gaps in service delivery by harnessing the resources and expertise of the private sector. However, it is crucial to strike a balance in designing incentives that attract private sector involvement while ensuring alignment with public health goals, transparency in partnerships, and equitable distribution of benefits to optimize the outcomes and impact of public–private collaborations in global health.

6.7 Data Reporting and Surveillance

In the realm of global health, incentivizing data reporting and surveillance plays a crucial role in strengthening public health systems. Health facilities and providers are incentivized to improve the reporting of disease outbreaks, health indicators, and other critical data by receiving benefits or recognition for their timely and accurate reporting. Incentives can take various forms, including financial rewards, access to additional resources or training, commendations, or accreditation (Custers et al., 2008). Timely and accurate reporting of health data is vital for early detection, rapid response, and effective control of disease outbreaks or health threats. When healthcare facilities and providers promptly report data, it enhances the capacity for robust surveillance systems, enabling public health authorities to track disease trends, identify emerging health concerns, and initiate timely interventions. Incentivizing data reporting not only fosters a culture of accountability and transparency within the healthcare system but also encourages adherence to reporting protocols, ultimately bolstering the accuracy and comprehensiveness of health information. However, it is essential to ensure that these incentives are structured in a way that encourages ethical reporting practices and does not compromise the integrity or quality of the reported data. Sustainable and equitable distribution of incentives, coupled with supportive mechanisms for data collection and reporting, are critical to fostering a robust and reliable global health surveillance infrastructure.

6.8 Sustainable Development

In the pursuit of sustainable development in the healthcare sector, incentives play a pivotal role in encouraging environmentally responsible health practices. One notable area where incentives are utilized is in promoting sustainability through initiatives aimed at reducing the environmental impact of healthcare facilities and operations. For instance, renewable energy initiatives within healthcare settings might receive incentives as a means to mitigate carbon footprints, decrease energy consumption, and foster environmentally-friendly practices (Rapport & Maffi, 2011). These incentives could come in various forms, such as tax credits, grants, subsidies, or preferential financing, which aim to offset the costs associated with implementing renewable energy sources like solar panels, wind turbines, or energy-efficient technologies in healthcare infrastructure. By incentivizing the adoption of sustainable energy practices, governments and institutions encourage the healthcare sector to embrace eco-friendly solutions, reducing reliance on fossil fuels, minimizing pollution, and contributing to overall environmental conservation efforts. Such initiatives not only promote sustainability within healthcare facilities but also serve as exemplars of responsible environmental stewardship within the broader context of global health. However, it is crucial that these incentives are structured and monitored effectively to ensure their viability, equitable distribution, and alignment with long-term sustainability goals in healthcare, emphasizing the importance of both environmental conservation and improved health outcomes.

7 In Summary: Incentives Used in Global Health Practices

It is imperative to acknowledge that while incentives wield potential effectiveness in specific contexts within global health practices, their design and implementation necessitate a cautious approach to mitigate unintended repercussions. Careful consideration should be given to crafting incentives that steer clear of unintended consequences, safeguarding against the compromise of fundamental principles such as equity, fairness, and the enduring sustainability of health initiatives. Striking a balance between incentivizing desired behaviors or outcomes and upholding ethical standards is crucial. This entails ensuring that incentives do not inadvertently exacerbate disparities or create inequitable access to healthcare resources. Moreover, prudent design should prevent potential short-term gains from undermining long-term goals, maintaining a steadfast focus on fostering sustainable and equitable improvements in global health practices. Therefore, while acknowledging their potential efficacy, the meticulous calibration of incentives remains pivotal to preserve ethical integrity and uphold equitable, sustainable health outcomes across diverse global contexts.

8 Profit from Humanitarian Crises

Humanitarian work is commonly linked with nonprofit organizations and dedicated individuals committed to delivering aid and support to vulnerable populations and communities facing crises or dire circumstances. The core mission of humanitarian efforts revolves around swiftly addressing pressing human suffering and mitigating the impacts of disasters, conflicts, and emergencies. The primary aim is to provide immediate relief, essential services, and critical assistance, focusing on alleviating hardship and restoring dignity to those affected by dire situations. Although the core of humanitarian work is grounded in altruism and the intent to aid others, there are scenarios where individuals might receive compensation or benefits tied to their engagement in such endeavors including salaries, consultation fees, living allowances, training and education, as well as recognition and awards.

8.1 Training and Education

In the field of humanitarian work, continuous learning and skill development are pivotal for workers to effectively respond to the evolving needs and challenges in providing aid and relief. Humanitarian organizations often provide their staff and volunteers with access to various training and educational opportunities aimed at enhancing their professional skills, knowledge, and competencies (Ottawa University, 2021). These opportunities encompass a wide array of areas, including emergency response, disaster management, healthcare delivery, logistics, cultural sensitivity, language proficiency, and more (Ottawa University, 2021). Participating in these training programs allows humanitarian workers to acquire new skills, deepen their expertise, and broaden their understanding of humanitarian principles and practices. Furthermore, these educational opportunities contribute to improving their readiness and adaptability in handling diverse situations and contexts during humanitarian operations (Ottawa University, 2021). The skills and knowledge gained from such training initiatives not only enhance workers' capabilities in their current roles but also bolster their qualifications and readiness for future career prospects within the humanitarian sector or related fields (Ottawa University, 2021). Thus, investing in training and education empowers humanitarian workers to become more effective, resilient, and versatile in providing assistance to communities in need.

8.2 Recognition and Awards

In the realm of humanitarian work, individuals and organizations engaged in exemplary efforts that significantly impact the lives of others may receive recognition, awards, or honors acknowledging their outstanding contributions. These accolades serve as affirmations of their dedication, innovation, and impactful interventions in addressing humanitarian crises or supporting vulnerable communities. Recognition and awards can take various forms, including prestigious honors from international organizations, governmental commendations, or awards from non-governmental entities specializing in humanitarianism. Such acknowledgments not only honor the commitment and achievements of individuals or organizations but also contribute to enhancing their personal or organizational reputation within the humanitarian community and beyond. The recognition received for outstanding humanitarian efforts often raises awareness about critical issues, inspires others to engage in similar initiatives, and fosters a positive image that may attract additional support or resources for future projects. Moreover, these awards serve as motivators, encouraging continued dedication and innovation in pursuing humanitarian causes and promoting positive change globally (WHO, 2023a).

It is imperative to underscore that while legitimate operational costs and compensations for workers are essential in the functioning of humanitarian organizations, profiteering or exploiting vulnerable populations stands in direct contradiction to the ethical principles guiding humanitarian endeavors. Esteemed humanitarian organizations prioritize transparency and accountability, ensuring that a significant portion of funding is allocated directly to providing aid and support for those most in need. Individuals engaged in humanitarian work typically exhibit a sincere dedication to assisting others, and their endeavors often yield positive, impactful outcomes for the individuals they aid. The benefits or compensations they receive are commonly regarded as a means to sustain their work and enable organizations to persist in their endeavors to serve affected communities.

9 Successful Initiatives

Throughout history, numerous impactful global health initiatives have demonstrated remarkable progress in enhancing public health and tackling specific health challenges on a worldwide scale. Below are several noteworthy examples of such initiatives, accompanied by their respective sources:

9.1 The Global Polio Eradication Initiative (GPEI)

GPEI is a partnership of various organizations, including WHO, UNICEF, Rotary International, the U.S. Centers for Disease Control and Prevention (CDC), and the Bill & Melinda Gates Foundation. It aims to eradicate polio globally through mass vaccination campaigns, surveillance, and community engagement. Since its launch in 1988, the number of polio cases has decreased significantly, with only a few countries still experiencing transmission (GPEI, n.d.).

9.2 Roll Back Malaria (RBM)

RBM is a global partnership launched in 1998 to combat malaria. It brings together governments, NGOs, businesses, and other stakeholders to coordinate efforts in malaria prevention, diagnosis, and treatment. RBM has contributed to substantial reductions in malaria-related deaths and infections in many high-burden countries (RBM, n.d.).

9.3 The Global Fund to Fight AIDS, Tuberculosis, and Malaria

The Global Fund is a financing mechanism that mobilizes resources to support programs against HIV/AIDS, tuberculosis, and malaria. It provides funding to countries to scale up prevention, treatment, and care services. Since its establishment in 2002, the Global Fund has saved millions of lives and played a crucial role in reducing the burden of these three major infectious diseases (The Global Fund to Fight, 2023).

9.4 Gavi, the Vaccine Alliance

Gavi is a public–private global health partnership that aims to increase access to vaccines in low-income countries. It supports immunization programs, facilitates the introduction of new vaccines, and negotiates lower vaccine prices. Gavi has contributed to significant progress in reducing vaccine-preventable diseases and improving vaccine coverage rates globally (Gavi, n.d.).

9.5 Partners in Health (PIH)

Partners in Health is a non-profit organization that provides healthcare services in resource-limited settings. They work to deliver high-quality medical care, strengthen health systems, and address social determinants of health. PIH's approach has shown success in improving health outcomes and reducing health disparities in several countries (Partners in Health, n.d.).

9.6 The STOP TB Partnership

The STOP TB Partnership is a global alliance working to eliminate tuberculosis (TB) as a public health problem. It facilitates collaboration among governments, civil society, and other partners to ensure universal access to TB diagnosis and treatment. Their efforts have contributed to progress in reducing TB incidence and mortality (UNOPS, n.d.).

10 Key Insights from These Successful Interventions

10.1 Multilateral Partnerships

The essence of multilateral partnerships lies in fostering collaboration and synergy among a spectrum of stakeholders, including governments, international organizations, non-governmental organizations (NGOs), private sector entities, and local communities (UN, 2019). This collaborative approach serves as a cornerstone for achieving substantive advancements in global health initiatives. These successful initiatives thrive on the collective efforts and diverse expertise brought forth by stakeholders working in unison towards shared objectives (UN, 2019). The beauty of such partnerships lies in leveraging the unique strengths, resources, and perspectives of each stakeholder, resulting in comprehensive, well-informed, and impactful strategies that address complex health challenges effectively (UN, 2019). This collaborative ecosystem fosters innovation, enables efficient resource utilization, and promotes inclusive decision-making, ultimately driving sustainable improvements in global health outcomes.

10.2 Global Solidarity and Commitment

These successful initiatives underscore the essence of concerted efforts and persistent commitment from nations, international bodies, and various stakeholders. Achieving meaningful progress in public health goals necessitates sustained dedication over extended periods, fortified by resolute political will and substantial financial support from the international community (WHO, 2023b).

Global solidarity, characterized by collaborative actions and unified endeavors across borders and sectors, plays a pivotal role. It encompasses mutual support, shared responsibilities, and collective action aimed at addressing common health challenges that transcend geographical boundaries (WHO, 2009). This solidarity fosters a sense of common purpose, encouraging nations and organizations to work hand-in-hand, pooling resources, expertise, and efforts toward achieving overarching public health objectives (WHO, 2009).

Moreover, the enduring commitment exhibited by governments, international agencies, philanthropic organizations, and other stakeholders remains critical. It involves prioritizing public health agendas, allocating sustained resources, and maintaining a steadfast focus on health outcomes, even amidst evolving global dynamics (WHO, 2023b). This steadfast commitment contributes to the continuity of initiatives, ensuring that efforts persist beyond immediate challenges, laying the groundwork for sustained improvements in global health on a long-term basis (WHO, 2023b).

10.3 Innovation and Research

The emphasis on innovation and research stands as a cornerstone in advancing global health initiatives, fostering breakthroughs in disease prevention and treatment modalities. Prioritizing research and innovation drives the development of novel technologies, methodologies, and interventions that significantly impact the landscape of public health (Perez & Ferretti, 2023).

Investment in research and development (R&D) forms the bedrock of progress in achieving global health objectives. It fuels the exploration of new scientific frontiers, fostering discoveries that can revolutionize disease prevention, diagnosis, and treatment (Perez & Ferretti, 2023). Robust R&D initiatives focus on uncovering effective vaccines, diagnostics, pharmaceuticals, and medical technologies essential in combating prevalent diseases and addressing emerging health threats (Perez & Ferretti, 2023).

Moreover, innovation sparks creative solutions to complex health challenges, fostering adaptability and responsiveness in the face of evolving health landscapes. Collaborations among scientists, healthcare professionals, academia, and industry leaders drive interdisciplinary approaches that catalyze breakthroughs, paving the way for transformative advancements in global health (Perez & Ferretti, 2023).

The commitment to research and innovation not only expands the horizons of medical knowledge but also cultivates a culture of continuous improvement and adaptation. It lays the groundwork for sustainable and impactful interventions, ultimately contributing to the enhancement of public health outcomes worldwide (Perez & Ferretti, 2023).

10.4 Targeted Interventions

Targeted interventions play a pivotal role in addressing specific health challenges, leveraging focused and evidence-based strategies to yield significant impacts. The essence of these interventions lies in their tailored nature, which involves customizing approaches to meet the distinct needs of diverse populations and contexts (Thornton et al., 2016).

By concentrating efforts on specific health challenges, targeted interventions maximize their effectiveness and efficiency. These initiatives are meticulously designed based on robust evidence, scientific research, and comprehensive data analysis (Thornton et al., 2016). They aim to pinpoint the root causes of health issues and implement interventions that directly address those underlying factors. This evidence-based approach ensures that resources, interventions, and strategies are precisely directed toward the most critical areas, optimizing their impact (Substance Abuse and Mental Health Services Administration [SAMSHA], 2022).

Moreover, tailoring interventions to suit the unique needs, cultural nuances, and contextual differences of different populations is imperative for success. By recognizing and accommodating diversity within communities, these interventions become more relevant, acceptable, and impactful (SAMSHA, 2022). Cultural competence and sensitivity in program design and implementation foster community engagement and participation, essential for the success and sustainability of interventions.

The flexibility inherent in targeted interventions allows for adaptability to changing circumstances, enabling rapid adjustments to meet evolving health challenges (SAMSHA, 2022). By focusing efforts on specific areas with tailored approaches, these interventions yield tangible and measurable results, contributing significantly to improving health outcomes in targeted populations (Thornton et al., 2016).

10.5 Holistic Approach

Successful initiatives in global health often adopt a holistic approach that extends beyond mere medical interventions, recognizing the intricate interplay between health and various social determinants. This holistic perspective acknowledges that health outcomes are influenced by a myriad of interconnected factors, including socio-economic, cultural, and environmental elements (Kumar & Preetha, 2012).

Addressing social determinants of health, such as poverty, education, nutrition, housing, access to clean water, gender equality, and social justice, is crucial in achieving comprehensive and sustainable improvements in health outcomes.

These determinants significantly impact an individual's health status, access to healthcare, and overall well-being (Kumar & Preetha, 2012). Hence, successful initiatives recognize the necessity of interventions that encompass broader social and environmental factors to create an enabling environment for better health.

By adopting a holistic approach, initiatives can tackle root causes rather than merely treating symptoms. For instance, addressing poverty through income generation programs or enhancing education opportunities can have a profound impact on health by empowering individuals and communities to access better healthcare, adopt healthier lifestyles, and make informed health-related decisions (Kumar & Preetha, 2012).

Moreover, promoting gender equality and social inclusion ensures equitable access to healthcare and opportunities for all, thus contributing to improved health outcomes for marginalized populations. Recognizing and addressing these multifaceted determinants create a more conducive environment that supports health and well-being at individual, community, and societal levels, fostering sustainable improvements in global health (Kumar & Preetha, 2012).

10.6 Data-Driven Decision Making

Data-driven decision-making is a cornerstone in successful global health initiatives, emphasizing the utilization of comprehensive and reliable data and evidence to guide informed decision-making processes. This approach involves systematic collection, analysis, and interpretation of data to derive actionable insights that shape strategies and interventions (Simon, 2023).

Robust monitoring and evaluation mechanisms are integral components of data-driven decision-making. These mechanisms enable continuous assessment of progress, identification of challenges, and adaptation of strategies in response to evolving circumstances (Simon, 2023). Through ongoing monitoring, initiatives can track key health indicators, measure the effectiveness of interventions, and identify areas requiring attention or improvement (School of Public Health, 2022).

The use of data and evidence facilitates the identification of trends, patterns, and gaps in healthcare delivery, enabling stakeholders to allocate resources efficiently and prioritize interventions based on identified needs (School of Public Health, 2022). Moreover, it fosters accountability and transparency within initiatives by providing measurable outcomes and benchmarks against which progress can be assessed (Simon, 2023).

By leveraging data-driven decision-making, initiatives can optimize their impact and effectiveness, ensuring that interventions are evidence-based, targeted, and responsive to the evolving health landscape. This approach empowers stakeholders to make informed choices, adapt strategies as necessary, and ultimately drive sustainable improvements in global health outcomes (School of Public Health, 2022).

10.7 Sustainability and Capacity Building

Sustainability and capacity building are integral components of successful global health initiatives, emphasizing the creation of lasting impacts and self-reliance within communities and healthcare systems. These initiatives prioritize strategies that not only address immediate health concerns but also empower local communities and healthcare workers to effectively manage and sustain their health outcomes in the long run (Kumar & Preetha, 2012).

Building local capacity involves empowering communities and healthcare workers with the knowledge, skills, resources, and infrastructure necessary to address health challenges independently. By providing training, education, and resources, initiatives enable communities to take ownership of their health, fostering a sense of self-sufficiency and resilience (Kumar & Preetha, 2012). Engaging communities in decision-making processes and involving them in the design and implementation of health programs enhances their sense of ownership, ensuring that interventions are culturally relevant, acceptable, and sustainable (Kumar & Preetha, 2012).

Moreover, strengthening health systems plays a crucial role in sustainability. Efforts directed toward improving infrastructure, healthcare delivery systems, access to essential medicines, and healthcare workforce development contribute to robust health systems. By enhancing the capacity and efficiency of health systems, initiatives ensure continued provision of quality healthcare services, even after the conclusion of specific programs or interventions (Kumar & Preetha, 2012). Promoting sustainability and capacity building fosters a legacy of self-reliance, resilience, and continued progress within communities and healthcare systems. Empowering communities to become active participants in their own health journey not only yields immediate benefits but also lays the groundwork for lasting improvements in global health outcomes (Kumar & Preetha, 2012).

10.8 Adaptability and Resilience

Adaptability and resilience serve as critical attributes in the realm of global health initiatives, recognizing the necessity of responding effectively to dynamic and evolving health challenges. These attributes enable initiatives to navigate uncertainties, address emerging health issues, and adjust strategies in a rapidly changing landscape (Blanchet et al., 2017).

In the context of global health, adaptability refers to the capability to modify approaches, strategies, and interventions in response to new information, emerging trends, or unforeseen circumstances. The ability to pivot and embrace innovative solutions when faced with unforeseen challenges ensures initiatives remain effective and relevant. Flexibility allows for the incorporation of new evidence, technology, or best practices, optimizing responses to complex health issues (Blanchet et al., 2017).

Resilience, on the other hand, pertains to the capacity to withstand and recover from setbacks, shocks, or adversities. Global health initiatives encounter multifaceted challenges, including disease outbreaks, natural disasters, socioeconomic changes, or geopolitical shifts (U.S. Agency for International Development [USAID], 2023). Resilience enables initiatives to endure these challenges, bounce back, and continue advancing their objectives despite obstacles. It involves building robust systems, fostering adaptable structures, and cultivating a culture of learning from experiences to fortify initiatives against future uncertainties (USAID, 2023).

Embracing adaptability and resilience ensures that global health initiatives remain agile and responsive, capable of addressing emerging health threats while enduring and overcoming obstacles. By integrating these qualities into their core strategies, initiatives can effectively navigate the complexities of global health, fostering sustainable and impactful outcomes amidst an ever-evolving landscape (USAID, 2023).

10.9 Equity and Access

Equity and access are fundamental pillars in successful global health initiatives, emphasizing fair and inclusive approaches to ensure that healthcare services and resources reach all individuals, particularly those who are vulnerable and marginalized (CDC, 2022a). These initiatives prioritize addressing health disparities and strive to create an environment where everyone has equal opportunities to attain good health and well-being (CDC, 2022b).

Health equity underscores the principle that everyone should have a fair opportunity to access healthcare services and resources needed to maintain good health, regardless of socio-economic status, geographic location, ethnicity, gender, or other determinants (CDC, 2022a, b). Successful initiatives proactively work to eliminate systemic barriers and inequities, aiming to provide equitable access to quality healthcare, essential medicines, preventive services, and health information (Global Health Council, 2022).

Moreover, these initiatives prioritize reaching marginalized and vulnerable populations, recognizing their increased susceptibility to health risks due to socio-economic, cultural, or geographical factors. By tailoring interventions to meet the specific needs of these populations, initiatives ensure that healthcare services are accessible, culturally sensitive, and inclusive, ultimately reducing health disparities (Global Health Council, 2022).

Addressing health disparities and promoting equity not only fosters social justice but also leads to improved overall health outcomes for entire communities and societies. By focusing on equitable access to healthcare and resources, successful initiatives strive to create a fairer and healthier world, where every individual, irrespective of their background, has the opportunity to lead a healthy life (CDC, 2022a).

10.10 Advocacy and Policy Influence

Advocacy and policy influence play pivotal roles in catalyzing transformative change in public health within global health initiatives. Engaging in advocacy efforts and influencing policies at various levels—local, national, and international—holds the potential to drive systemic and sustainable improvements in public health outcomes (Wilson et al., 2023).

Advocacy efforts within global health initiatives involve raising awareness, mobilizing stakeholders, and voicing concerns to address health-related challenges. These efforts aim to garner support, galvanize public opinion, and drive action toward health priorities. Advocacy can take diverse forms, such as campaigns, community engagement, or coalition-building, and is geared toward influencing policymakers, decision-makers, and key stakeholders to prioritize health issues (Wilson et al., 2023).

Influencing policies is a key strategy in effecting enduring change. Policies, laws, and regulations shape the landscape of public health by determining resource allocation, healthcare delivery systems, access to services, and health promotion initiatives. Advocacy efforts focused on influencing policy seek to advocate for evidence-based policies that support health and well-being, ensure equitable access to healthcare, and address systemic barriers that hinder optimal health outcomes (Wilson et al., 2023).

Moreover, successful global health initiatives recognize the interconnectedness between health and various sectors, such as education, environment, and economy. Engaging in policy advocacy allows initiatives to bridge health-related gaps across sectors, fostering comprehensive and integrated approaches that promote overall well-being (Wilson et al., 2023).

By engaging in advocacy and influencing policies, global health initiatives can effectuate systemic changes that drive sustainable improvements in public health. Policies that prioritize health and well-being contribute significantly to the creation of healthier communities and societies, ensuring that populations have access to essential healthcare services and conducive environments that support optimal health (Wilson et al., 2023).

These key points underscore the significance of collaborative efforts, grounded in evidence-based approaches, and the adoption of a far-sighted outlook within global health initiatives. Drawing insights from successful endeavors and implementing these learnings enables the global health community to consistently propel forward, making substantial strides in mitigating health challenges and enhancing the welfare of individuals across the globe.

References

Abduljawad, A., & Al-Assaf, A. F. (2011). Incentives for better performance in health care. *Sultan Qaboos University Medical Journal, 11*(2), 201–206.

Abimbola, S., & Topp, S. M. (2018). Adaptation with robustness: The case for clarity on the use of 'resilience'in health systems and global health. *BMJ Global Health, 3*(1), e000758.

Banati, P., & Moatti, J. P. (2008). The positive contributions of global health initiatives. *Bulletin of the World Health Organization, 86*(11), 820. https://doi.org/10.2471/blt.07.049361

Blanchet, K., Nam, S. L., Ramalingam, B., & Pozo-Martin, F. (2017). Governance and capacity to manage resilience of health systems: Towards a new conceptual framework. *International Journal of Health Policy and Management, 6*(8), 431–435. https://doi.org/10.15171/ijhpm.2017.36

Braveman, P. A., Kumanyika, S., Fielding, J., LaVeist, T., Borrell, L. N., Manderscheid, R., & Troutman, A. (2011). Health disparities and health equity: The issue is justice. *American Journal of Public Health, 101*(S1), S149–S155.

Brown, L., LaFond, A., & Macintyre, K. (2001). *Measuring Capacity Building*. University of North Carolina at Chapel Hill.

Center for Disease Control and Prevention. (2021). *Global Health Equity Strategy 2022–2027*. December 16, 2023, https://www.cdc.gov/globalhealth/equity/pdf/globalhealthequity.pdf

Centers for Disease Control and Prevention. (1999). *The Principles of Disease Elimination and Eradication*. Centers for Disease Control and Prevention. https://www.cdc.gov/mmwr/preview/mmwrhtml/su48a7.htm

Centers for Disease Control and Prevention. (2021, October 20). *Cost-effectiveness analysis*. Centers for Disease Control and Prevention. https://www.cdc.gov/policy/polaris/economics/cost-effectiveness/index.html

Centers for Disease Control and Prevention. (2022a, December 2). *Vision for Health Equity in CDC's global work*. Centers for Disease Control and Prevention. https://www.cdc.gov/globalhealth/equity/vision.html

Centers for Disease Control and Prevention. (2022b, December 2). *Vision for Health Equity in CDC's global work*. Centers for Disease Control and Prevention. https://www.cdc.gov/globalhealth/equity/vision.html

Clements, B. W., & Casani, J. (2016). *Disasters and public health: Planning and response*. Butterworth-Heinemann.

Cooper, A. (2016). *Governing global health: Challenge, response, innovation*. Routledge.

Custers, T., Hurley, J., Klazinga, N. S., & Brown, A. D. (2008). Selecting effective incentive structures in health care: A decision framework to support health care purchasers in finding the right incentives to drive performance. *BMC Health Services Research, 8*(1), 1–14.

Durrance-Bagale, A., Marzouk, M., Tung, L. S., Agarwal, S., Aribou, Z. M., Ibrahim, N. B. M., Mkhallalati, H., Newaz, S., Omar, M., Ung, M., Zaseela, A., Nagashima-Hayashi, M., & Howard, N. (2022). Community engagement in health systems interventions and research in conflict-affected countries: A scoping review of approaches. *Global Health Action, 15*(1), 2074131. https://doi.org/10.1080/16549716.2022.2074131

Global Polio Eradication Initiative. GPEI. (n.d.). https://polioeradication.org/

Gavi. (n.d.). The Vaccine Alliance. http://www.gavi.org/

Glanz, K. (1997). *Theory at a glance: A guide for health promotion practice* (No. 97). US Department of Health and Human Services, Public Health Service, National Institutes of Health, National Cancer Institute.

Global Health Council. (2022, August 29). *Four pillars part 3: Global Health Equity*. Four Pillars Part 3: https://globalhealth.org/four-pillars-part-3-global-health-equity/

Haldane, V., Chuah, F. L. H., Srivastava, A., Singh, S. R., Koh, G. C. H., Seng, C. K., & Legido-Quigley, H. (2019). Community participation in health services development, implementation, and evaluation: A systematic review of empowerment, health, community, and process outcomes. *PLoS ONE, 14*(5), e0216112. https://doi.org/10.1371/journal.pone.0216112

Injustice Has a Cure. Partners in Health. (n.d.). http://www.pih.org/
Kumar, S., & Preetha, G. (2012). Health promotion: An effective tool for global health. *Indian Journal of Community Medicine: Official Publication of Indian Association of Preventive Social Medicine, 37*(1), 5–12. https://doi.org/10.4103/0970-0218.94009
Murray, C. J., & Frenk, J. (2000). A framework for assessing the performance of health systems. *Bulletin of the World Health Organization, 78*, 717–731.
Ottawa University. (2021, January 12). *Why is Training and Development Important?* https://www.ottawa.edu/online-and-evening/blog/january-2021/5-benefits-of-training-and-development
Pan American Health Organization, & World Health Organization. (n.d.). *Health Indicators Conceptual and Operational Considerations.*
Perez-Aleman, P., & Ferretti, T. (2023). Creating innovation capabilities for improving global health: Inventing technology for neglected tropical diseases in Brazil. *Journal of International Business Policy, 6*(1), 84–114. https://doi.org/10.1057/s42214-022-00143-y
Pierson, L., & Verguet, S. (2023). When should global health actors prioritise more uncertain interventions? *The Lancet. Global Health, 11*(4), e615–e622. https://doi.org/10.1016/S2214-109X(23)00055-4
Rapport, D. J., & Maffi, L. (2011). Eco-cultural health, global health, and sustainability. *Ecological Research, 26*(6), 1039–1049.
RBM Partnership to End Malaria. (n.d.). https://endmalaria.org/
School of Public Health. (2022). *Data-driven decision-making for Health Administrators*. Tulane University School of Public Health. (2022, December 22). https://publichealth.tulane.edu/blog/data-driven-decision-making/
Schorr, L., Farrow, F., & Sparrow, J. (2014, November). *An evidence framework to improve results.* In Harold Richman Public Policy Symposium, Center for the Study of Social Policy.
Simon, B. (2023, September 6). *Data-Driven Decision-Making: The Missing Piece in Development Projects*. USAID Learning Lab. https://usaidlearninglab.org/community/blog/data-driven-decision-making-missing-piece-development-projects
Substance Abuse and Mental Health Services Administration. (2022). *Community Engagement: An Essential Component of an Effective and Equitable Substance Use Prevention System.* Substance Abuse and Mental Health Services Administration.
The Global Fund to Fight AIDS, Tuberculosis and Malaria. (2023). http://www.theglobalfund.org/
The Commonwealth Fund. (n.d.). *Public Programs Are Using Incentives to Promote Healthy Behavior*. https://www.commonwealthfund.org/publications/newsletter-article/public-programs-are-using-incentives-promote-healthy-behavior#:~:text=Using%20incentives%20to%20change%20unhealthy,active%20role%20in%20their%20care.
Thornton, R. L., Glover, C. M., Cené, C. W., Glik, D. C., Henderson, J. A., & Williams, D. R. (2016). Evaluating strategies for reducing health disparities by addressing the social determinants of health. *Health Affairs Project Hope, 35*(8), 1416–1423. https://doi.org/10.1377/hlthaff.2015.1357
Trouiller, P., Olliaro, P., Torreele, E., Orbinski, J., Laing, R., & Ford, N. (2002). Drug development for neglected diseases: A deficient market and a public-health policy failure. *The Lancet, 359*(9324), 2188–2194.
United Nations. (2019). *United Nations Sustainable Development Cooperation Framework.*
UNOPS. (n.d.). Stop TB Partnership. https://www.stoptb.org/
USAID. (2023). *Promoting Resilience*. U.S. Agency for International Development. (2023, March 10). https://www.usaid.gov/global-health/health-systems-innovation/health-systems/promoting-resilience
WHO Commission on Social Determinants of Health, & World Health Organization. (2008). *Closing the gap in a generation: health equity through action on the social determinants of health: Commission on Social Determinants of Health final report.* World Health Organization.
WHO. (2009, June 22). *Why the World Needs Global Health Initiatives*. World Health Organization. https://www.who.int/director-general/speeches/detail/why-the-world-needs-global-health-initiatives

WHO. (2023b, September 12). *Unprecedented Focus on Global Public Health at UN General Assembly*. World Health Organization. https://www.who.int/news/item/12-09-2023-WHO-urges-focus-on-health-goals-at-UN-General-Assembly

WHO. (2023a, May). *Public health prizes and awards*. World Health Organization. https://apps.who.int/gb/awards/

Wilson, L., Hamwi, S., Zanni, F., & Lomazzi, M. (2023). Global public health policies: Gathering public health associations' perspectives. *Global Health Action, 16*(1), 2183596. https://doi.org/10.1080/16549716.2023.2183596

World Economic Forum. (2023) *Global Health and Healthcare Strategic Outlook: Shaping the Future of Health and Healthcare*.

World Health Organization. (n.d.). *Social Determinants of Health*. World Health Organization. https://www.who.int/health-topics/social-determinants-of-health#tab=tab_1

Yang, A., Farmer, P. E., & McGahan, A. M. (2010). Sustainability' in global health. *Global Public Health, 5*(2), 129–135. https://doi.org/10.1080/17441690903418977

12 Challenges and Solutions to the Sustainability of Humanitarian Activities in Burkina Faso

Namara R. Swillum

Abstract

The Sahel region faces several hazards that necessitate humanitarian action, including armed conflict, destabilized governments, violent extremism and climate change. The environment shaped by these elements in the region presents barriers to sustainable, adequate and efficient humanitarian activities. In the context of Burkina Faso, humanitarian relief services conducted by the government and civil society organizations (CSOs) alike face these challenges and more, including barriers to financial stability, capacity building, and security of land resources. Challenges associated with financial stability in Burkina Faso are linked to issues in the international humanitarian funding structure and over-prioritization of select needs. Difficulties in capacity building while linked to financial instability, also involves under-recognition leading to a limitation in networking opportunities. Securing land resources for use in Burkina Faso has had varying results due to differences in resource management design, implementation and upkeep. This chapter highlights humanitarian activities in Burkina Faso led by both the government and CSOs to alleviate conditions brought on by regional and country-specific issues and what barriers they are working against. Solutions offered by scholars are discussed and dissected for their feasibility in strengthening the continuity of humanitarian operations in Burkina Faso. Additional context-informed solutions are presented; the results call for International non-governmental organizations (INGOs) to re-evaluate their role in humanitarian activities. Upon reviewal, Burkina Faso's government needs to expand infrastructure development activities to address previously

N. R. Swillum (✉)
College of Public Health, University of South Florida, Tamp, FL, USA
e-mail: namara@usf.edu; namaraswillum@gmail.com

S. Spowart (ed.), *Global Happiness and Humanitarian Assistance*, Integrated Science 29, https://doi.org/10.1007/978-3-031-71789-5_12

failed projects. Increased partnership with CSO in humanitarian activities is necessary and recognition of the progress made due to their involvement should not be understated.

Keywords

Community health workers • Telecommunications • Agricultural development • Networking • Complex humanitarian crises

1 Challenges and Solutions to the Sustainability of Humanitarian Activities in Burkina Faso

Burkina Faso resides in the region of Sahel, an area represented in various articles assessing the context of humanitarian aid activities during armed conflict. Both Dieng (2021) and Ferraro (2021) assess barriers in connecting vulnerable populations to humanitarian services and finds weak governance and armed conflict in the Sahel region to be primary sources. Understanding the surrounding geography of Burkina Faso and associated challenges within the region is essential in the process of recognizing barriers and solutions to sustaining humanitarian activities in the country because of how these concerns transcend borders and perpetuate the continued violence in Burkina Faso. This paper aims to establish the cross-border regional context of challenges that limit governmental and civil society organizations (CSOs) in their capacities to provide sustainable humanitarian assistance in the Sahel region. From there, barriers specific to the conditions in Burkina Faso can be identified and reviewed for how they might negatively interact with region-wide challenges. This assessment corresponds with relevant solutions presented in literature, which are then discussed and understood for their feasibility in promoting the continuation of humanitarian provisions in Burkina Faso.

2 The Sahel Regional Context

As aforementioned the Sahel, a region comprising of ten countries beginning at the Atlantic Ocean and stretching to the Red Sea while nested between the Sahara Desert and the savannas, is subject to armed conflict and weak governance, in addition to violent extremism, and climate change (Dieng, 2021; Ferrar, 2021). Armed conflict presents a challenge to the sustainability of humanitarian initiatives in the region because of continued international humanitarian law (IHL) violations from both state and non-state groups; these conditions have increased security concerns and prevented safe allocation and distribution of humanitarian services (Dieng, 2021; Ferrar, 2021). The presence of terrorism within the armed groups active in the region increase the prevalence of sporadic deadly attacks and spillovers from neighboring countries (Dieng, 2021).

The national governments present in the region, including Burkina Faso, are susceptible to stakeholder pressures and are often unable to safeguard their citizens from the atrocities their own military forces commit (Dieng, 2021; Ferraro, 2021). To enact the protections of humanitarian providers in the landscape, state and non-state groups must agree to not disrupt or harm humanitarian intervention and be able to reasonably ensure this; humanitarian services already on the ground continue to be cut off from resources and unable to reach areas with the most vulnerable populations (Coppola, 2020; Dieng, 2021; International Committee of the Red Cross [ICRC], 2022). This is especially the case in Central Sahel, where Burkina Faso is located; attacks against citizens by both armed groups and security forces have been ethnically and religiously motivated due to their identity's association with community defense groups (Dieng, 2021). This, combined with the disruption of education and targeting of children during violence, adds to the list of challenges needing to be addressed through humanitarian, and legal, avenues (Dieng, 2021). These attacks on civilians and civilian objects have led to increased environmental degradation of land used by pastoralists and farmers in Sahel, a region already vulnerable to climate change (Dieng, 2021).

Climate change is presented as challenge to the Sahel region as a whole rather than just Burkina Faso because of the intra-state effects of violence on land quality and the reality that climate change does not obey borders. Conflict, by acting as a physical barrier to land and water usage and a polluter, in collaboration with scarce resources as a result of climate change, has forced the movement of persons and land-use (Dieng, 2021). Pastoralists seek better land for their cattle to graze upon and farms seek safer, healthier ground to grow their crops on (Dieng, 2021). As a result, they have increasingly crossed paths, leading to violent battles over land rights and competition for resources (Dieng, 2021). Their land-usage rights conflict has been co-opted by terrorist groups in an effort to recruit new members (Dieng, 2021). The violence, scarce resources, and extreme events increased by climate change strain the capacity of humanitarian organizations in the region to serve their communities by limiting safe passageways, sources of supplies, and increasing public health risks (Dieng, 2021). Everyone is trying to escape the violence, but not even refugee camps can offer protections to displaced persons due to a total disregard of IHL by state and non-state groups involved in the conflict (Dieng, 2021). Burkina Faso is not alone in the challenges they face, but it is because their neighboring states are facing a similar reality.

Various countries in the region attempt to impose protections for humanitarian organizations to function within to provide essential aid via the provision of armed escorts or declaring state of emergencies to limit potential activities of armed groups in the area (Ferraro, 2021). However, this puts humanitarian providers in a position where their protections granted under IHL are at risk of being violated due to their proximity with security forces, and their movements being restricted (Coppola, 2020; Ferraro, 2021). Governmental humanitarian initiatives also find themselves trapped in this association with military forces, making their own interventions inherently risky (Ferrar, 2021). In the context of Sahel, armed protection invites violence and puts humanitarian workers and assets at further risk of harm

(Ferraro, 2021). This is the environment that humanitarians in Burkina Faso work within to address the needs of at-risk populations.

3 Challenges and Solutions in Burkina Faso

There are multiple constraints that threaten the sustainability of governmental and CSO initiatives that vary in the type of humanitarian services they provide. Primarily providing healthcare interventions to civilians in Burkina Faso, both CSOs and government workers face several barriers to financial stability and increasing capacities in ways that ultimately support the continuation of community led initiatives and partnerships. Financial barriers are primarily represented in the regional discourse about Global North international NGOs (INGOs) dominance in the region and country outshining community needs, as well as the recognition that the government of Burkina Faso simply does not have the means to increase funding. Barriers to capacity building at CSOs is extensively represented through the limits of current infrastructure, and stakeholder networking. Challenges associated with the security of land resources are discussed independently from these topics because they provide an opportunity to analyze why globally supported solutions to water scarcity and food insecurity have seen both success and failure in Burkina Faso.

3.1 Financial Stability

The presence of Global North international NGOs (INGOs) in Burkina Faso is arguable as much as a barrier as it is a benefit in providing humanitarian services to Burkina Faso. Kumi and Yeboah (2021) collected statements from several CSOs staff members in various countries, including Burkina Faso, about their perception of the role INGOs in aid localizations. Aid localization is the utilization of empowering communities and other CSOs to collaborate on the sustainability of CSOs and identify local networking, partnerships and supply chain access in their respective communities (Kumi & Yeboah, 2021). Regional stakeholders representing CSOs disagree about whether the presence of INGOs in aid localization is colonial because aid localization is a concept INGOs came up with to organize CSOs, or because aid localization was established by CSOs and INGOs are now co-opting the movement and claiming credit (Kumi & Yeboah, 2021). In either case, there is an agreement among regional CSOs that the presence of INGOs in this concept is a continuation of colonial practices in the humanitarian sector that lead to INGOs with greater power in the field (Kumi & Yeboah, 2021). At the same time CSOs in the region recognize that they benefit when INGOs allocate funds to distribute directly to them; however, CSOs argue that without INGO presence in the area, humanitarian donors could focus their attention and funding towards local CSOs who are better equipped to understand the needs of their community than INGOs (Kumi & Yeboah, 2021).

For healthcare workers in Burkina Faso, they see the role that INGOs can play with country governments to market one specific priority need so much that another is unaddressed simply because of unawareness about provided services (Samuelsen, 2020). For example, Samuelson (2020) noted that the marketing of the fight against malaria created a supply–demand nexus in Burkina Faso where community members sought health services for predominately malaria screening because they knew that is what their local health services offered, rather than seeking health services in general or for other services offered but not as advertised as malaria. This can produce unintended consequences for a community when other health concerns may begin to arise prior to national and international attention (Samuelsen, 2020). Additionally, it can leave little funding budgeted for other community needs, leaving other responses without funding (Samuelsen, 2020).

3.1.1 Solutions

Solutions to the financial dependency on INGOs as presented in the results of surveys by Kumi and Yeboah (2021): INGOs need to be guided towards ant-colonial practices that aim to uplift humanitarian activities of national and local CSOs and government programs. These practices include the facilitation of coordination and collaboration that is CSO, or government led, listening and adhering to needs stipulated by community-based organizations rather than trying to reframe what their humanitarian services they offer to accommodate INGO priorities (Kumi & Yeboah, 2021). One interviewee describes this process as creating allies between both Global North and Global South organizations (Kumi & Yeboah, 2021). Another stated that INGOs and international donors need to stop stereotyping CSOs as being unable to appropriately utilize funds; in turn, CSOs need to commit to transparency and accountability to promote an environment where they can be trusted with stable funding (Kumi & Yeboah, 2021). A solution to the context of over-advocacy hiding other priority needs and thus limiting financial stability for corresponding strategies and initiatives, has to be based around a willingness of INGOs and government partners to create feedback loops. This would allow CSOs and governmental humanitarian workers to give feedback that is actively considered and supported as appropriate. As such, current marketing methods for initiatives can be reviewed for changes and allocation funding and resources can be reassessed.

3.2 Capacity Building

Rural areas of Burkina Faso lack sufficient infrastructure that supports access to electricity and telecommunication systems and poses as a challenge to increasing use of digital technologies to address health concerns and provide telehealth services to vulnerable populations (Arnaert et al., 2019). Despite this, mobile health (mhealth) remains a supported solution to limited access to healthcare because it can be overcome by travelling to a town with access to such infrastructure to charge devices and make the appointments (Arnaert et al., 2019). In one case, the presence of a phone for mhealth services in a village provided access for the whole community to health services, thus extending humanitarian services digitally to all of them (Arnaert et al., 2019).

In the sector of humanitarian assistance for emergency education and child well-being interventions, a lack of social networking and fostering partnerships within the abundant field of humanitarian actors is seen as a challenge to their activities (Balbone et al., 2022). Their lack of linkage to projects can indicate their activeness in the field; Balbone et al.'s (2022) study revealed that although some Sahel and Burkina Faso based CSOs ranked low in achievements, they are associated with being primary contributors to emergency education and child protections response activities. The study also reveals the lack of recognized partnerships by large INGOs and that several of them and UN agencies fail to consider local actors they work with as part of their network of stakeholders (Balbone et al., 2022). This can limit CSOs and decentralized government initiatives from receiving recognition and resources that increase their capacity to serve civilians in Burkina Faso.

3.2.1 Solutions

The situation of infrastructure is improving thanks to the strengthening capacities of the Burkina Faso government in improving technological infrastructure and increasing access country-wide (Arnaert et al., 2019). Arnaert et al. (2019) argues that the introduction of mhealth in isolated regions will increase the sustainability of services there once infrastructure projects are complete. Similar to the solution of creating financial stability through allyship with INGOs, CSOs need to continue to advocate for their recognition as equal partners in the humanitarian field. This is something the Burkina Faso government has the capacity to help them with and support their recognition as part of the stakeholder network.

3.3 Security of Land Resources

As briefly aforementioned, conflict and climate has led to the damage and destruction of farmers' fields across the Sahel region, and the movement of people seeking better land. In conjunction with the degradation of the environment and displacement, the issue of water scarcity and food insecurity became exacerbated (Somda et al., 2020; World Food Programme [WFP], 2023). There are several methods that have already been implemented by both the government of Burkina Faso and non-governmental organizations to overcome these challenges and improve food security and water access across the country, including agricultural development in inland valleys and training-based food security programs to engage community members in food production and nutritional healthcare (Baki et al., 2022; Wilson et al., 2023; Yacouba et al., 2019). It is important to note that agricultural development is widely seen as an effective humanitarian method to combat food insecurity and reduce the amount of water used in agricultural production, thereby increasing water availability for consumption (Food and Agricultural Organization [FAO], n.d.; Pawlak & Kołodziejczak, 2020).

However, not all interventions have been as successful as they could be. Barriers to the success of agricultural developments coordinated by the government for use by small time farmers is uncovered in two separate studies, one conducted by Yacouba et al. (2019), and the other by Somda et al. (2020). Wilson et al. (2023) provides information about barriers to sustaining community-based worker (CBW) projects in Burkina Faso after facilitating organizations complete their exit strategy. Despite challenges, utilizing food security projects that rely on CBWs as a method to support food production and water conservation in inland valley agricultural developments has the potential to increase the incorporation of sustainable farming practices and organize farmers enough to grow their production capacities and lose less water.

3.3.1 Challenges to Sustaining Agricultural Development

The Burkinabe government began investing in the agricultural development of inland valleys and uplands in the 1970s to counter the severe drought's impact on water availability for consumption and increase agricultural yields sustainably to improve outcomes for their civilians (Baki et al., 2022; Yacouba et al., 2019). Inland valleys are identified as a solution to reduce the impact of climate change because they are typically water-rich due to their seasonal transformation into flooded wetlands and have nutrient rich soils that provide a reliable environment for farming and water catchment (Somda et al., 2020). By the 2000s, the shift towards agricultural production in these areas became a method of enhancing food security and reducing poverty, as these developments were utilized by local farmers supporting rural communities (Baki et al., 2022). Two methods have been used to harness the natural landscape of inland valleys in Burkina Faso: (1) small reservoirs with irrigation systems; and (2) bunds and canals (Somda et al., 2020; Yacouba et al., 2019).

In the case of reservoirs, many are dated and in disrepair, impairing the capability of local food production and water conservation activities (Somda et al., 2020). Through various assessments of water infrastructure in Burkina Faso, it was found in some locations that the design of reservoirs were impeded by poor water management planning due to lack of historical data on the local environment's hydrological cycle (Somda et al., 2020). Their sustainability was also hampered by poor upkeep and maintenance after construction (Somda et al., 2020). Further, the varying practices of farmers continues to limit growth in agricultural production in Moutori and Fafo, both locations relying on small reservoirs (Somda et al., 2020). Moutori farmers experience greater losses of water during irrigation than Fafo, despite irrigating less frequently (Somda et al., 2020). Despite these challenges, the implementation of reservoirs in Burkina Faso are seen as largely successful due to higher yields, increased sustainability of food production and improved water control in the agricultural sector (Somda et al., 2020).

3.3.2 Solutions

Both types of agricultural development in Burkina Faso can see improved water control and agricultural production through increased maintenance and further development. For reservoirs, this entails finding ways to reduce surface evaporation, organizing farmers, and mobilizing outside organizations and government agencies to provide support and maintenance services (Somba et al., 2020). Specific to the situation in the BIV, more drainage flumes need to be installed in locations supported by extensive topographic surveys of the area (Yacouba et al., 2019). The waterlogging can be further reduced via digging canals; however, this might increase the risk of erosion in the valley and over-drain the landscape if not adequately analyzed for such risks (Yacouba et al., 2019). Given that both reservoir-supported and bund and canal system agricultural developments are utilized by a multitude of independent farmers, they would both likely benefit from learning about sustainable farming practices and how they can be implemented within their own practices to grow food production and improve water conservation. Somba et al. (2020) suggested farmers organize, however did not indicate how this solution could be implemented. The issue of farmers using varying practices hampering food production and water control could be solved through the incorporation of food security projects based in training residents to be CBWs for their communities; this practice by non-governmental organizations entails training farmers to train each other in sustainable farming techniques (Wilson et al., 2023). There are challenges in continuing CBW programs after facilitating organizations withdraw, but they can be further studied and organizations can help create more sustainable networks and identify resource allocation sources to support continuation (Wilson et al., 2023).

4 Discussion

Solutions presented by scholars are offered by civilians of Burkina Faso and the Sahel region who are keenly aware of the ongoing violence. Other solutions, as suggested by this paper, are informed by an understanding of the complex humanitarian crisis that overlaps borders in the Sahel region and create the environment that Burkina Faso CSOs and governmental programs operate within to support their communities. Capacity building for Burkina Faso organizations can be difficult when populations in the region continue to be displaced and migrate away from violence. However, the government, as seen focusing projects of technological infrastructure and even in investment of their health services, show how they are responding to barriers and finding ways they can improve conditions and increase the agency of civilians. It is important to note that the focus on technological advancement should not prevent the appropriate financing and updating of water infrastructure for agricultural development and implementation of sustainable farming techniques. Child protection groups are an important part of humanitarian activities in Burkina Faso because of the active recruitment of young boys into armed group forces and violence against adolescent girls across the Sahel region (Balbone et al., 2022; Dieng, 2021).

INGOs, particularly Global North ones, are revealed as contributing to problems faced during humanitarian activities of local, national and regional CSOs and governments. They are seen as organizations that distract donors from funding on the ground, community led humanitarian aid (Kumi & Yeboah, 2021). In the same way they distract donors towards their concerns, INGOs distract vulnerable populations from understanding that their health services are more than just opportunities to screen for malaria (Samuelsen, 2020). Likewise, funding is allocated to INGO concerns rather than needs identified by CSOs and government initiatives. Yet, this turmoil with the involvement of INGOs cannot negate the need for their recognition and involvement in stakeholder networks and financial stability of CSOs and government programs (Balbone et al., 2022; Kumi & Yeboah, 2021). These elements increase capability building processes that are essential for the sustainability of humanitarian activities in Burkina Faso.

5 Conclusion

The Sahel region is faced with armed conflict complicated by terrorists, armed groups, weak state governance, and climate change; the unfortunate reality is that climate change in the region increases violence of those concerned about land rights. All of this violence creates an environment in the region where humanitarian action is restricted by their ability to traverse the landscape and put their own lives at risk or disobey state declaration of emergencies by governing officials. Armed escorts are not a solution to safeguarding humanitarian aid because it makes the application of IHL protections difficult. Within Burkina Faso, CSOs and government programs traverse the realities of their security crisis with barriers in securing financial stability and increasing their capacities to account for displaced populations and new situations that arrive within the complex climate. Technology is seen as a solution, as well as collaboration coordination through the use of stakeholder networks. Local actors need to be recognized by their INGO constituents as active members of their network. INGOs must continue to turn away from colonial practices in humanitarian aid and ensure that communities lead planning and implementation. Further, the upkeep of water infrastructure in inland valley agricultural zones must be prioritized, in addition to community mobilized education of farmers working the land on sustainable farming techniques. The lack of maintenance, adequate planning and advancement of agricultural development in inland valleys in Burkina Faso has limited overall food production and water conservation efforts and, in some cases, has led to abandonment of developments that could be salvaged.

References

Arnaert, A. L., Ponzoni, N., Debe, Z., Meda, M. M., Nama, N. G., & Arnaert, S. (2019). Experiences of midwives and community health workers using mHealth to improve services to pregnant women in rural Burkina Faso, Africa. *Journal of Nursing Education and Practice, 10*(3), 57–64. https://doi.org/10.5430/jnep.v10n3p57

Baki, C. B., Wellens, J., Traoré, F., Palé, S., Djaby, B., Bambara, A., Thao, N. T. T., Hié, M., & Tychon, B. (2022). Assessment of hydro-agricultural infrastructures in Burkina Faso by using multiple correspondence analysis approach. *Sustainability, 14*(20), 13303. https://doi.org/10.3390/su142013303

Balbone, A., Sieza, Y., & Naboho, N. (2022). Coming together? Social network analysis of humanitarian actors in Burkina Faso. *The Humanitarian Leader.* https://doi.org/10.21153/thl2022art1574

Coppola, D. (2020). *Introduction to International Disaster Management* (Ed. 4). Butterworth-Heinemann.

Dieng, A. (2021). The sahel: Challenges and opportunities. *International Review of the Red Cross, 103*(918), 765–779. https://doi.org/10.1017/S1816383122000339

Djagba, J. F., Rodenburg, J., Zwart, S. J., Houndagba, C. J., & Kiepe, P. (2014). Failure and success factors of irrigation system developments: A case study from the Ouémé and Zou Valleys in Benin. *Irrigation and Drainage, 63*(3), 328–339. https://doi.org/10.1002/ird.1794

Ferraro, R. (2021). Challenges to implementation of humanitarian access norms in the Sahel. *International Review of the Red Cross, 103*(918), 859–882. https://doi.org/10.1017/S18163831220 0025X

Food and Agriculture Organization [FAO]. (n.d.). *Water Management.* https://www.fao.org/land-water/water/water-management/en/

International Committee of the Red Cross [ICRC] (2022, February). *After Ten Years of Armed Violence in the Sahel, There is Still Time for Humanity* [Statement]. https://www.icrc.org/en/document/after-ten-years-armed-violence-sahel-there-still-time-humanity

Kumi, E. K., & Yeboah, T. Y. (2021). Localisation agenda, shift the power and African philanthropic models in Burkina Faso, Ghana, Nigeria and Senegal. *West Africa Civil Society Institute (WACSI).* https://doi.org/10.15868/socialsector.39047

Pawlak, K., & Kołodziejczak, M. (2020). The role of agriculture in ensuring food security in developing countries: Considerations in the context of the problem of sustainable food production. *Sustainability, 12*(13), 5488. https://doi.org/10.3390/su12135488

Samuelsen, H. (2020). Accelerated fragility: Exploring the supply–demand nexus in health facilities in rural Burkina Faso. *Africa, 90*(5), 934–951. https://doi.org/10.1017/S00019720200 00662

Somda, W., Tischbein, B., & Bogardi, J. J. (2020). Water use inside inland valleys agro-systems in the Dano basin, Burkina Faso. *Water Cycle, 1*, 88–97. https://doi.org/10.1016/j.watcyc.2020.06.003

UN Guiding Principles Reporting Framework. (n.d.). *Civil Society Organizations (CSOs).* https://www.ungpreporting.org/glossary/civil-society-organizations-csos/

Wilson, K. R., Rogers, B. L., Carroll, D. A., Ezaki, A., & Coates, J. (2023). Sustainability of community-based workers in multisectoral food security programs: A case study of producer leaders, village vaccinators, mother leaders, and community health workers in Burkina Faso. *Agriculture & Food Security, 12*, 30. https://doi.org/10.1186/s40066-023-00432-6

World Food Programme [WFP]. (2023, October). *WFP Burkina Faso Country Brief*. https://docs.wfp.org/api/documents/WFP-0000154992/download/?_ga=2.263581068.1488446353.1703985081-545063659.1703985080

Yacouba, Y., Aymar, B. Y., Amadou, K., Louis, F. J., Georges, S., Thomas, Y. B., Mouhamed, I., & Bruno, L. (2019). Failure of inland valleys development: A hydrological diagnosis of the Bankandi Valley in Burkina Faso. *Modeling Earth Systems and Environment, 5*, 1733–1741. https://doi.org/10.1007/s40808-019-00628-5

Haiti: Understanding Humanitarian Assistance in Conflict

13

Juliet Winther

Abstract

Haiti's ongoing humanitarian crisis is marked by severe political instability, economic decline, and recurrent natural disasters. This paper works to understand the multifaceted nature of the situation in Haiti, including its historical context, current socio-economic and health challenges, and the impact of violence and human rights violations. Despite significant international aid, the crisis has worsened due to persistent gang violence, extreme poverty, and failing infrastructure. This paper further explores the effectiveness of humanitarian responses, such as the influence of the Sphere Handbook's standards and community engagement practices, while highlighting the limitations and ethical concerns faced by aid organizations. Understanding the crisis in Haiti can lead to further enhancing security measures for humanitarian workers, an increase in funding, and improving community resilience. This paper highlights the urgent need for a coordinated, comprehensive approach to address both immediate needs and long-term recovery in Haiti.

Keywords

Haiti • Humanitarian assistance • Conflict • Gang activity • International aid

There are numerous instances that may necessitate the provision of humanitarian assistance to meet the critical needs of the vulnerable populations affected. While humanitarians are known to respond to a broad network of emergencies,

J. Winther (✉)
CPH Provisional, College of Public Health, University of South Florida, 13201 Bruce B. Downs Blvd, MDC 56, Tampa, FL 33612, USA
e-mail: juliet7@usf.edu

S. Spowart (ed.), *Global Happiness and Humanitarian Assistance*, Integrated Science 29, https://doi.org/10.1007/978-3-031-71789-5_13

some of the most common humanitarian crises may range from natural disasters, armed conflicts, and epidemics to widespread poverty, displacement, and food insecurity. Haiti, one of the most populated countries in the Caribbean, continues to be affected by a deteriorating humanitarian crisis put into place by continued instances of political gridlock, economic recession, inflation, and escalating violence (Office for the Coordination of Humanitarian Affairs [OCHA], 2023a). Additionally, Haitian citizens continue to face the adverse effects of environmental emergencies, such as the devastating earthquake that struck Haiti in 2010 (United States Geological Survey, 2011). Following the 2010 earthquake, Haiti also experienced several severe weather events due to the worsening climate crisis, including two hurricanes that shook the country and regular flooding due to increased rainfall in the region (World Bank, 2021).

1 History of Haitian Crisis

The humanitarian crisis in Haiti is preceded by a troubled, and violent history. Over the course of several centuries, the Haitian population has enduringly grappled with the consequences of violence and conflict, deeply rooted in the historical legacies of slavery and colonization. Prior to Haitian independence in 1804, the region was faced with several colonization attempts from countries such as Spain and later France (United States Department of State, n.d.). Despite Haiti's initial independence in 1804, Haitian independence wasn't officially recognized by the United States until 1862 (United States Department of State, n.d.), Following several successful efforts to gain independence, political instability and violent uprisings continue to leave Haiti in a desperate humanitarian crisis. Most recently, following the assassination of President Jovenel Moise, the region has experienced increasing inflation and unemployment, leading to approximately 90% of Haitans living below the poverty line, while a third live in extreme poverty (OCHA, 2023d). This fragile state was only furthered by Haiti's high prevalence of severe weather events, such as earthquakes, hurricanes, and flooding. Haitian Health.

2 Demographics

The worsening situation in Haiti is accompanied by a significant rate of communicable and noncommunicable diseases within the population. According to the Pan American Health Organization, noncommunicable diseases continue to be one of the leading causes of death and disease burden within Haiti (Pan American Health Organization [PAHO], 2021). The region boasts some of the highest rates of mortality by noncommunicable diseases, as well as high rates of disability-adjusted life years (PAHO, 2021). High rates of noncommunicable diseases such as hypertension, obesity, and diabetes continue to present issues for an already overwhelmed health system (PAHO, 2021). Similarly, there are several prevalent communicable diseases found in Haiti. Some of the most common diseases reported include tuberculosis, HIV, malaria, and dengue fever (PAHO, 2021).

3 Haiti Humanitarian Crisis

Over the past decade, the humanitarian crisis in Haiti has continued to significantly deteriorate. High rates of unemployment and a severe lack of resources and a lack of skilled workers has led to severe poverty in the region (Pierre, 2020). While education is viewed in Haiti as an influential factor to ending poverty, many families cannot afford to send their children to school, fostering generational poverty and an economic downturn (Pierre, 2020). Additionally, as armed groups continue to perpetuate violence against Haitian citizens, public health professionals are seeing a significant increase in human rights violations, including kidnapping, lynching as well as sexual and gender-based violence against women, girls and boys (OCHA, 2023b). In 2022, Haiti reported approximately 16,500 incidents of gender-based violence, including physical, sexual, and emotional violence (Office for the Coordination of Humanitarian Affairs [OCHA], 2023c). Increasing rates of gang-violence and general conflict, has further led to a desperate need for humanitarian assistance in Haiti (OCHA, 2023c). According to the Office for the Coordination of Human Affairs (OCHA), there are more than 300 gangs present in the region, with influential actions varying from political reasons to security interests (OCHA, 2023d). This is furthered by the fact that more than 200,000 Haitian individuals may be experiencing internal displacement due to violence or poor community infrastructure, with almost half reporting precarious or inadequate shelter conditions (OCHA, 2023b).

In the wake of the 2010 earthquake that struck Haiti, a devastating cholera outbreak rapidly spread across the region. According to the Centers of Disease Control and Prevention (CDC), there were approximately 400,000 cases of cholera reported between 2011 and 2019 (Centers for Disease Control and Prevention [CDC], 2023). Additionally, as of October 2022, a new cholera outbreak is beginning to ravage the country, with over 600 confirmed- and 7,000 suspected- cases reported (CDC, 2023). According to the Office for the Coordination of Humanitarian Affairs, more than half of Haiti's population is in need of humanitarian assistance; this may include services dedicated to food, water, shelter, sanitation, health, and psychosocial support (OCHA, 2023b). In addition to the assistance required due to increased rates of violence, the humanitarian crisis was only furthered as the consequences of COVID-19 continued to ravage the globe.

Haiti has also fallen victims to several severe weather events, in addition to the 2010 earthquake. Due to Haiti's position in the Atlantic Ocean, the region is especially vulnerable to hurricanes. In October of 2016, a category 4 hurricane struck Haiti, destroying the majority of homes throughout the region, and injuring or affecting upwards of 2 million individuals (Marcelin et al., 2017). Long-term consequences of this hurricane included a decrease in food production, lack of accessible and safe shelters, lack of access to safe drinking water, and overall destruction of the country's agricultural sector (Marcelin et al., 2017). Communities in Haiti may also experience increased flooding, due to the low-lying nature of many Haitian regions.

Even as Haiti continues to experience conflict after conflict, the Haitian government remains passive in the face of violence and human rights violations. Despite the existence of some of the worst human rights violations in history, the Government of Haiti refuses to identify and prosecute the individuals and groups most responsible (United States Department of State, 2022). Human rights violations are not only seen at the hand of armed groups and through gang violence, but also at the hands of Haitian authorities. In addition to overwhelming reports of the police force's denial of assistance and care, many individuals have reported abuse at the hands of police, and other local authority figures (Lanham et al., 2019).

4 Protection of Human Rights: Problems and Solutions

Human rights violations are regularly seen during times of conflict, and the region of Haiti is no exception. According to the United States Department of State, human rights organizations in Haiti have been reporting high rates of kidnapping, food deprivation, physical and sexual violence, and other forms of abuse across the region (United States Department of State, 2022). Additionally, social isolation due to fear and gang presence prevents those affected from seeking healthcare, or necessary resources. While multiple international governmental and non-governmental organizations have released statements condemning the human rights violations in Haiti, there has yet to be an effective policy to decrease the prevalence of these violations.

While millions of individuals across Haiti continue to experience human rights violations, certain populations are more vulnerable. Women and girls continue to experience gender-based violence (GBV) at a significantly higher rate than men and boys. In addition to women and girls, other vulnerable groups include lesbian, gay, bisexual, transgender, queer, and intersex individuals (United States Department of State, 2022). According to the United Nations Population Fund, approximately 64% of those experiencing GBV are women, while approximately 33% are girls (United States Agency for International Development [USAID] 2023). While types of GBV vary, there are several common forms seen in Haiti. Individuals in Haiti may experience GBV in the form of intimate partner violence (IPV), sexual violence, femicide, human trafficking, female genital mutilation (FGM), and child marriages (United Nations, 2023). Thus, women and girls are being disproportionately affected by the human rights violations occurring in Haiti.

5 Key Humanitarian Frameworks

There are several humanitarian frameworks that professionals should implement in the case of a humanitarian crisis such as the one currently faced by Haiti. While the core humanitarian principles may be useful in this case due to its overall violent and political nature, the standards set by the Sphere Handbook is the more comprehensive framework. It sets the expectations for humanitarian response in four sectors; water supply and sanitation, food security and nutrition, shelter and settlement, and health (OCHA, 2018). Given the comprehensive scope and severity of the situation in Haiti, the utilization of Sphere standards may present an opportunity for humanitarian actors to devise targeted assistance programs aimed at mitigating the detrimental impacts of the crisis.

Additionally, the implementation of community engagement practices may aid in the sustainability of the programs put in place by humanitarian aid. Through local empowerment and an overall strengthening of local capabilities, humanitarians can ensure that the approaches are culturally and traditionally sensitive. The incorporation of local knowledge and perspectives will also aid in the development of contextually appropriate implementations. Similarly, through the participation of influential and respected community leaders, community members will see these programs as credible and reliable. This will aid in a sense of legitimacy and trust among the community, which will lead to the effectiveness of the overall approach.

Overall, community engagement practices may pave the way for future growth, development, and recovery following this humanitarian crisis. Allowing for a stronger sense of community engagement will also provide for a continued evaluation, as community engagement fosters a sense of open dialogue. This will allow for consistent updates and modifications of these programs received through those most affected by the programs. Additionally, open dialogue will aid in the de-stigmatization of gender, sex, and race hopefully leading to reduced rates of human rights violations.

A cluster approach may also be successful in the Haitian crisis. This approach aims to further the coordination and cooperation between the different sectors of humanitarian response, while continuously maintaining accepted humanitarian standards (Dhillon et al., 2012). A cluster approach will allow humanitarian workers in Haiti to approach the situation through joint collaboration between stakeholders and humanitarian workers. Through this, humanitarians are able to target stakeholders' main concerns, and develop programs and resources to best assist the most vulnerable populations. Finally, humanitarian workers should consider implementing the Do No Harm approach. This will minimize any negative humanitarian action through not worsening the conflict, and it will also discourage local dependency on humanitarian workers (Khaled, 2021).

6 Actors and Stakeholders

In order to create a comprehensive humanitarian strategy, understanding the needs of stakeholders is crucial. Due to the complex nature of the crisis in Haiti, there are many stakeholders to consider, both locally and internationally. Local stakeholders include the national and local administrative sectors, civil society, churches, and local communities. In this case, the local stakeholders would include the Government of Haiti, local communities in Haiti, and Haiti's private sector, including but not limited to, businesses, companies, and crisis response. International stakeholders may include donors, media, international governmental organizations, and international non-governmental organizations (NGOs). There are several paths that humanitarians can take to fully understand and validate the concerns of these individuals and groups. Qualitative methods such as surveys, questionnaires, and focus groups will allow for a better understanding of the stakeholder's primary concerns. As previously mentioned, including influential community figures will also allow for a sense of community involvement in the project, ensuring that the needs of the community are met in addition to the needs of the financial stakeholders.

7 Humanitarian Response

Many organizations have sent assistance to combat the worsening crisis in Haiti. International governmental and non-governmental institutions, such as the United Nations and the United States Department of International Aid, have provided assistance by sending essential resources and funding, such as emergency food and healthcare supplies and approximately $206 million in financial assistance (United States Agency for International Development [USAID], 2023). They have also deployed Disaster Assistance Response Teams to assist with the situation, and implemented training and education programs within the affected areas (USAID, 2023). These training programs are primarily focused on the following; good hygiene practices, safe drinking water, and the strengthening of Haitian healthcare systems to respond to past and future pandemics (USAID, 2023). Additionally, the 2023 Haiti Humanitarian Response Plan noted several planned improvements to aid in the recovery and sustainability of Haiti. Within this plan, the Office for the Coordination of Humanitarian Affairs highlighted significant changes within the Haitian agriculture sector that may help to improve the worsening food insecurity (OCHA, 2023c). This program also sets targets for health, nutrition, child protection, education, and water sanitation, among several other sectors (OCHA, 2023c).

Several other groups have also sent resources and humanitarian teams to assist with the crisis in Haiti. From international organizations such as Doctors without Borders, to smaller more local organizations such as the Haitian Health Foundation, there are hundreds of organizations working to aid the crisis in Haiti. While these organizations continue to make significant strides in combating the challenges in Haiti, there is still room for improvement in the humanitarian sector.

Due to the traumatic nature of the situation, organizations should offer mental health and emotional counseling services to combat the stresses faced by individuals across the nation. A 2019 study showed that 86% of adults in four key Haitian neighborhoods reported either moderate or severe psychological distress (Tymejczyk et al., 2019). Additionally, psychological stress was seemingly more prevalent among women and girls (Tymejczyk et al., 2019). While this could be due to a number of factors including a genetic disposition to mental health issues, societal factors such as the prevalence of gang violence, increasing gender-based violence and kidnappings may have a startling influence on this trend.

As the conflict in Haiti worsens, humanitarian efforts have been growing and changing to accommodate the unpredictable landscape. However, studies have shown that the humanitarian sector may not be growing fast enough to accommodate the volume of need. A 2023 survey revealed that only a small fraction of aid has been received in Haiti, and the aid that was given did not cover priority needs among affected individuals (Stoddard et al., 2023). The survey also demonstrated a lack of humanitarian presence, and accessibility issues due to a lack of knowledge and transportation to where aid was being provided (Stoddard et al., 2023).

8 Challenges and Ethical Considerations

When establishing a humanitarian plan, there are several challenges and ethical considerations that must be taken into consideration. A study done in 2019 highlighted three major complications faced by humanitarians. These challenges include providing the highest attainable quality of care, protecting workers, and minimizing unintended harms (Broussard et al., 2019). Due to the complex and violent nature of many humanitarian crises, it is crucial that humanitarian organizations take worker safety into account. In humanitarian work, especially in regions affected by conflict, humanitarian health workers are at risk of general violence and direct attacks, which may result in severe injuries or death (Broussard et al., 2019). According to the United Nations, approximately 62 humanitarian workers have been killed as of August, 2023.

(United Nations, 2023). Similarly, 84 workers have been wounded, while 34 have been kidnapped (United Nations, 2023). Additionally, this danger also presents adverse consequences for humanitarians such as psychological harm, economic loss, and interruption of services (Broussard et al., 2019). Violence against humanitarian workers continues to be a major hurdle in providing safe and efficient humanitarian assistance. This violence may lead to the immediate dismissal of humanitarians, even in situations where it is most needed. Thus, the problems faced by humanitarian workers can indirectly affect individuals in affected regions through the suspension of essential services not found anywhere else.

Conflict settings may also present several ethical challenges unique to humanitarian work. Due to a shortage of necessary resources and personnel, humanitarian health workers may be forced to practice outside of their scope of training, which is a severe health ethics violation (Broussard et al., 2019). A lack of required resources may leave patients untreated, due to the need to triage those most at risk, creating a gap in healthcare access among individuals in the affected area (Broussard et al., 2019). In a crisis setting, humanitarian organizations may also be faced with ethical considerations regarding rebuilding destroyed structures, where to focus special attention, and stakeholder risk. Additionally, as stated in the humanitarian frameworks, it is crucial that humanitarian organizations stay neutral, even with the demands of involved parties and international and domestic donors hanging over their heads.

9 Socio-Economic Impact

Due to the continued conflict and political instability in Haiti, professionals continue to see adverse consequences on the socioeconomic status of millions of individuals across the region. High rates of financial insecurity have led to Haiti being considered the poorest country in the Caribbean, and amongst the poorest in the world by economic professionals (The World Bank, 2023). According to UNICEF, approximately 59% of the Haitian population lives below the poverty line, while approximately 24% live in extreme poverty (UNICEF, 2023). Additionally, Haiti continues to rank 163 out of 191 regions on the 2021 Human Development Index (UNICEF, 2023). High poverty rates often present adverse consequences among affected regions and individuals.

Consequences of low socio-economic status may lead to poor mental, physical and emotional health. This is due to several factors, including a lack of access to healthcare. A 2021 study demonstrates that less than 10% of the Haitian population have access to health insurance (Cenat et al., 2021). The country also lacks a comprehensive mental health care system due to a severe lack of psychiatrists, psychologists and social workers to care for a population of over 11 million individuals (Cenat et al., 2021). Haiti's poor socioeconomic status may also be to blame for a lack of overall development, as this region is considered to be the least advanced in the Latin American and Caribbean region (Economic Commission for Latin America and the Caribbean [ECLAC], 2013). Socio-economic factors in this region continue to hinder the recovery and humanitarian efforts within Haiti.

10 Proposed Solutions

Despite humanitarian efforts to reduce the suffering in Haiti, the conflict continues to worsen. While domestic and international organizations continue to offer relief in the form of funding and the provision of basic resources, more work is needed to further aid the situation. While several international governments have provided monetary support to aid in the rebuilding of the region, significantly more funding is needed. Organizations such as the United Nations International Children's Fund are desperately requesting more funding in order to keep up with the growing number of individuals requiring humanitarian assistance (United Nations International Children's Fund [UNICEF], 2021). In order to ensure that the money is actually being used to implement the institution reforms necessary for Haiti to recover, it is crucial that the money is directed to non-governmental organizations assisting in Haiti. The United States government is also working to improve the Haitian government accountability, in hopes this will improve quality of life in Haiti (United States Government Accountability Office, 2023). Additionally, the development of several risk reduction implementations may protect individuals in the case of emergency evacuations for weather, conflict, or health. Through the development of early warning systems, public health and disaster management specialists will be able to initiate an effective and timely evacuation in case of severe weather events, high levels of conflict or violence, or during epidemics and/or pandemics. The development of community resilience strategies may also aid in the risk reduction for future emergencies.

To ensure the safety and well-being of humanitarian workers engaged in the crisis response, as well as to enhance the sustainability and effectiveness of the humanitarian response plan in Haiti, it is important to prioritize and significantly enhance worker safety and security measures. This can be done through the implementation of a sector dedicated solely to worker safety. This sector should be solely responsible for providing safe and secure spaces for humanitarians, as well as the provision of security personnel, whether it is paid guards, or through the United States military. Additionally, welfare checks should be done regularly to assess the physical and mental health and well-being of humanitarian workers in the field. This will help ensure the longevity and efficacy of this program, as workers will not be dismissed or sent home for safety or health reasons. To further enhance the ethics of humanitarian action in Haiti, an ethical review board should be established. By having a team of ethical professionals involved in critical decision-making processes, the humanitarian sector can ensure that ethical considerations are thoroughly examined and integrated into the decision-making framework. This will then allow for increased transparency, accountability, and integrity within the humanitarian efforts undertaken in Haiti.

11 Limitations

While the proposed solutions may seem relatively straight forward, there are several things to consider. Developers of these proposals may notice several strengths or limitations in the plan, which may lead to necessary modifications. Funding continues to be one of the defining factors of Haiti's recovery. However, many humanitarian organizations are reporting a severe lack of funding. According to the United Nations, its World Food Program (WFP) has only received 16% of the funding required to further assist Haiti, leaving approximately $121 million left (United Nations, 2021). This demonstrates a lack of available emergency funds across the globe, without which the program may not be able to continue.

Additionally, this proposal may be halted due to infrastructural and environmental factors. Haiti's primary infrastructure, which is an important aspect of distributing resources and deploying personnel, is oftentimes inadequate or even completely inaccessible (United Nations, n.d.). This may prevent necessary resources from reaching communities most affected, as they may be blocked off due to collapsed buildings and roads. This further limits the humanitarian workers' access to remote areas, which already presented a problem due to Haiti's rugged terrain and isolated regions.

The proposed safety and security implementations may present several unique limitations. As tensions in this region worsen, less and less individuals may want to work in the humanitarian field. Thus, leading to a shrinking workforce. Consequences of this may include inadequate personnel for the proposed improvement in security and safety measures. Funding may play a significant part here as well, as humanitarian organizations may lack the necessary funding to pay security risk management professionals. Without adequate safety measures, humanitarians may begin to see a decline in the labor force. This will only harm the proposed interventions by decreasing rates of necessary personnel by significant rates. A lack of adequate collaboration between stakeholders and humanitarian workers may also hinder the process. In the past, the Haitian Government has been at the forefront of major corruption cases (United States Department of State, 2022). This may show to be an issue during the implementation of programs. A lack of cooperation from local and federal agencies will be detrimental to the growth of the proposal, as well as to the recovery of Haiti as a whole.

12 Past Humanitarian Successes

Despite the worsening conditions in Haiti, there is still hope for recovery. According to the Pan American Health Organization, humanitarian efforts in Haiti have been successful in several sectors. Essential medical supplies and treatment is being increasingly offered across the region, specifically targeting victims of human rights violation and gender-based violence (Pan American Health Organization [PAHO], 2021). While there needs to be a significant improvement in funding for this crisis, available funds have aided in the strengthening and emergency response of communities in Haiti (European Commission, 2023). Following the 2010 cholera epidemic, high levels of funding from governmental organizations, such as the European Commission, allowed for the resources and personnel needed to reach the eventual decline of the pandemic (European Commission, 2023). The implementations proposed only seek to further the achievements humanitarian workers have already made in Haiti. Additionally, this program seeks to reach the majority of affected individuals, instead of a small portion as previously demonstrated.

13 Conclusion

This paper has demonstrated the severity of the humanitarian crisis that is currently affecting Haiti. While humanitarian efforts are vast, and focused on many different sectors, the situation continues to worsen. Factors like political instability, gang violence, and human rights violations continue to persist across the region, leading to adverse conditions for the Haitian population. This situation demonstrates the need for enhanced humanitarian response efforts, and a significant need for emergency funding. Governmental and non-governmental organizations should continue to work on the public condemnation of violence and human rights violations, while also providing assistance through resources, training programs, and funding.

Conflicts of interest This paper has never been presented, there are no conflicts of interest.

References

Broussard, G., Rubenstein, L. S., Robinson, C., Maziak, W., Gilbert, S. Z., & DeCamp, M. (2019). Challenges to ethical obligations and humanitarian principles in conflict settings: A systematic review. *Journal of International Humanitarian Action*. https://doi.org/10.1186/s41018-019-0063-x

Cenat, J. M., Harerimana, B., Michel, G., McIntee, S. E., Mukunzi, J. N., Hajizadeh, S., & Dalexis, R. D. (2021). The global challenge of providing mental health services in poverty: the situation of Northern Haiti. *Cambridge University Press*. https://doi.org/10.1192/bji.2021.22

Centers for Disease Control and Prevention (CDC) (2023, 25 January). *Cholera in Haiti*. https://www.cdc.gov/cholera/haiti/index.html

Dhillon, P., & Annunziata, G. (2012, 5 September). The Haitian health cluster experience: A comparative evaluation of the professional communication response to the 2010 earthquake and the subsequent cholera outbreak. *PLOS Currents*. 10.1371%2F5014b1b407653

Economic Commission for Latin America and the Caribbean (ECLAC) (2013, January). *Social protection systems in Latin America and the Caribbean: Haiti*. https://www.cepal.org/en/publications/4075-social-protection-systems-latin-america-andcaribbean-haiti

European Commission (2023). *Cholera in Haiti*. europa.eu

Khaled, A. F. (2021). Do no harm in refugee humanitarian aid: the case of the Rohingya humanitarian response. *Journal of International Humanitarian Action*. https://doi.org/10.1186/s41018-021-00093-9

Lanham, M., Ridgeway, K., Dayton, R., Castillo, B.M., Brennan, C., Davis, D.A., Emmanuel, D., Morales, G.J., Cheririser, C., Rodriguez, B., Cooke, J., Santi, K., & Evens, E. (2019, March 11) We're going to leave you for last, because of how you are: Transgender women's experiences of gender-based violence in healthcare, education, and police encounters in latin America and the Caribbean. https://doi.org/10.1089/vio.2018.0015

Marcelin, L. H., Cela, T., & Shultz, J. M. (2017). Haiti and the politics of governance and community responses to Hurricane Matthew. *Disaster Health*. https://doi.org/10.1080/21665044.2016.1263539

Office for the Coordination of Humanitarian Affairs (OCHA) (2023a, 7 September). *Haïti Health Cluster: Navigating a Multifaceted Humanitarian Crisis*. https://reliefweb.int/report/haiti/humanitarian-community-haiti-deeply-concerned-about-continued-escalation-violence

Office for the Coordination of Humanitarian Affairs (OCHA) (2023b, 31 August). The humanitarian community in Haiti is deeply concerned about the continued escalation of violence. https://reliefweb.int/report/haiti/humanitarian-community-haiti-deeply concerned-about-continued-escalation-violence

Office for the Coordination of Humanitarian Affairs (OCHA) (2023c, 13 April). Haiti: humanitarian response plan 2023 at a glance. https://reliefweb.int/report/haiti/haitihumanitarian-response-plan-2023-glance-april-2023-enht

Pan American Health Organization (PAHO) (2021). *Country Profile: Haiti.* https://hia.paho.org/en/countries-22/haiti-country-profile

Pierre, G. R. (2020). Poverty in Haiti. *Open Journal of Political Science.* https://doi.org/10.4236/ojps.2020.103025

Stoddard, A., Harvey, P., Duque-Diez, M., Czwarno, M., & Breckenridge, M.J. (2023, August). Humanitarian access SCORE report: Haiti. *Humanitarian Outcomes.* https://www.humanitarianoutcomes.org/publications/score-report-Haiti-2023

Transgender Women's Experiences of Gender-Based Violence in Healthcare, Education, and Police Encounters in Latin America and the Caribbean. *Violence and Gender.* https://doi.org/10.1089/vio.2018.0015

The World Bank (2023). *The World Bank in Haiti.* https://www.worldbank.org/en/country/haiti/overview#:~:text=Haiti's%20economic%20nd%20social%20development,poorest%20countries%20in%20the%20world

Tymejczyk, O., Rivera, V. R., Peck, M., Dorelien, A., Petion, J. S., Seo, G., Walsh, K. F., Pape, J. W., McNairy, M. L., Fitzgerald, D. W., Nash, D., & Parcesepe, A. (2019, November 23). Psychological distress among a population-representative sample of residents of four slum neighborhoods in Port-au-Prince, Haiti. HHS Public Access. 10.1016%2Fj.jad.2019.11.103

United Nations (2021). *WFP forced to slash food aid as half of all Haitians go hungry.* https://news.un.org/en/story/2023/07/1138787#:~:text=Severe%20shortfall,the%20end20of%20the%20year

United States Department of State (2022). *Major Corruption Cases in Haiti and Government of Haiti.* https://www.state.gov/wp-content/uploads/2022/11/Appendix-C-Developments-inHaiti-004977.pdf

United States Agency for International Development (USAID) (2023, November). *Haiti.* https://www.usaid.gov/humanitarian-assistance/haiti

United Nations (2023a). *FAQs: Types of violence against women and girls.* https://www.unwomen.org/en/what-we-do/ending-violence-against-women/faqs/types-of-violence

United Nations (2023b). *20 years after deadly attack on UN in Iraq, humanitarian workers remain committed to help, #NoMatterWhat, despite growing risks.* https://www.unocha.org/news/20-years-after-deadly-attack-un-iraq-humanitarian-workers-remain-committed-help-nomatterwhat

United States Department of State (n.d.). *A Guide to the United States' History of Recognition, Diplomatic, and Consular Relations, by Country, since 1776: Haiti.* https://history.state.gov/countries/haiti

U.S. Geological Survey (usgs.gov). (2011). Overview of the 2010 Haiti earthquake. *Overview of the 2010 Haiti Earthquake Earthquake Spectra, 27*(1_suppl1), 1–21. https://doi.org/10.1193/1.3630129

Overview and Summary Conclusion 14

Sara Spowart

Abstract

This book provides an investigation of numerous aspects related to global happiness and humanitarian assistance. There are multiple sections to this book including 1) high-level overviews, 2) topics related to special and vulnerable populations, and 3) case study explorations in different countries. An evaluation of problems, potential solutions, and trends for the future are explored throughout this book.

Keywords

Global happiness • Humanitarian assistance • Innovation • Case studies • Special populations

This book covers a multitude of topics related to global happiness and humanitarian assistance. Some key points include a global overview of the topic and understanding in the early chapters. Then the second part includes an exploration of large-scale humanitarian issues as well as accompanying solutions. The third part explores issues related to special populations in humanitarian assistance situations such as refugees, women, children, and individuals with mental illness. The final part of the book explores case study examples and solution-oriented interventions for humanitarian situations such as in Haiti, Syria, and Burkina Faso. The book is meant to provide a large-scale overview of global happiness, issues with

S. Spowart (✉)
College of Public Health, University of South Florida, Tampa, USA
e-mail: compassionbasedhappiness@gmail.com; sara.spowart@gmail.com

S. Spowart (ed.), *Global Happiness and Humanitarian Assistance*, Integrated Science 29, https://doi.org/10.1007/978-3-031-71789-5_14

solutions, special populations, and case study examples. It points to the significance of incorporating happiness into the humanitarian assistance agenda as well as practical interventions to make this feasible.

The manufacturer's authorised representative in the EU is Springer Nature Customer Service Centre GmbH, Europaplatz 3, 69115 Heidelberg, Germany. If you have any concerns regarding our products, please contact ProductSafety@springernature.com

Printed and bound by CPI Group (UK) Ltd, Croydon, CR0 4YY
30/09/2026
02225584-0002